I0048585

Home Tube Feeding: A mini casebook

Also by the author:

Your Tube: A guide to nutrition through a feeding tube

Home Tube Feeding

A mini casebook

LINA BREIK

Advanced Accredited Practising Dietitian

First published 2024

Copyright © Lina Breik 2024

The moral rights of the author have been asserted.

All rights are reserved, except as permitted under the
Australian Copyright Act 1968 (for example, fair dealing for
the purposes of study, research, criticism or review). No
part of this book may be reproduced, stored in a retrieval
system, communicated or transmitted in any form or by any
means without prior written permission from the author.

Typesetting by BookPOD
Cover illustration by Paul Telling © The visual storytellers
group 2024 – www.visstorytellers.com.au

ISBN: 978-0-6459873-2-4 (pbk)
ISBN: 978-0-6459873-3-1 (e-book)

NATIONAL
LIBRARY
OF AUSTRALIA

A catalogue record for this
book is available from the
National Library of Australia

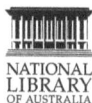

"Embracing the challenge of providing nourishment through a feeding tube is not just within our dietetic capabilities; it is another opportunity to showcase the transformative impact we can have on lives as dietitians."

Lina Breik

"Now why am I writing about this in the first place? Because so many people don't understand it. Every day my radar picks up subtle signs of people who wonder what the deal is. How do I eat and drink? What's going on? Do I actually have a tube going into my stomach? Yes, and they do too. It's in their throats."

Roger Ebert, Tube-Fed Film Critic (1942–2013)

Contents

Introduction

Welcome to this mini casebook on home tube feeding!

Inside, you'll find 20 clinical cases, each paired with insightful commentary, inspired by the real-life experiences of individuals managing feeding tubes at home.

Whether you're a student or an experienced dietitian, this casebook is designed to support you. These cases aim to empower you to adopt a person-centred, evidence-based approach while also encouraging you to think creatively when faced with complex situations.

Each case begins with a brief background outlining the primary issue at hand, followed by commentaries (not answers!) on potential interventions and investigations to address the issue. It concludes with notes (or references) and further reading recommendations, as well as reflective questions to consider post-case.

To keep the content accessible, each case is concise, focusing on one specific issue related to home tube feeding. The omission of detailed social, medical, and nutritional histories reflects the reality that home care clinicians often work with limited information. This brevity is intentional, allowing you to focus on key issues without feeling overwhelmed.

Before you begin, here are a few important points to consider:

► *There is no one-size-fits-all solution.* The 'right' approach for each of these cases often depends on the preferences of the individual with the feeding tube (even if these preferences deviate from standard practices). The challenge – and beauty – of healthcare is accommodating these preferences while ensuring clinical safety.

► *The commentaries are not exhaustive.* They are meant to stimulate critical thinking rather than offer all-encompassing solutions (which would be impossible anyway!).

► *Collaborative learning is invaluable.* Working through the cases with a peer, mentee, mentor, or in a tutorial group setting will expose you to diverse perspectives, enriching your learning experience. Post-case reflective questions follow each case to foster interaction and encourage real-world application.

► This casebook takes a unique approach *by not focusing on routine calorie and protein calculations.* Instead, it encourages you to go beyond the basics in supporting adults with home tube feeding.

▶ Please note that this book is *intended as a learning tool, not as a clinical practice guideline* or direct clinical advice for individuals with feeding tubes.

I encourage you to reflect on each case, considering the unique needs and preferences of the individuals you may encounter. Use these scenarios to think critically, engage with research, and develop personalised care plans. The goal is to enhance your problem-solving skills and deepen your understanding of home tube feeding management.

Please remember, while these cases are inspired by real experiences, they have been de-identified, and the names, social situations, medical diagnoses, and ages have been altered. Any resemblance to actual persons or situations is purely coincidental.

Thank you for choosing this casebook to expand your knowledge of home tube feeding. Wishing you happy learning and the best of luck in your practice!

Passionate about making a difference,

Lina Breik

Jen – Sudden Bowel Movement Changes

Jen is a 27-year-old woman who sustained a traumatic brain injury following a motor vehicle accident when she was 18. Jen lives with her older sister, and they love going out for social outings together, such as seeing a movie or going to a café.

Jen currently weighs 50 kilograms (kg), while her ideal body weight is 53 kg. She has a radiologically inserted gastrostomy (RIG), size 18 French (Fr), with the external skin disc or flange positioned at 2.5 centimetres (cm) at skin level.

Regarding her nutrition, Jen receives 200 millilitres (ml) of a 1.5 kilocalorie (kcal)/ml formula at 0630, 0930, 1230 and 1830. Additionally, she enjoys an oral snack of sliced avocado and yoghurt at 1530. She also has 50 ml of water before and after each bolus feed, along with an extra 100 ml water flush at 1100, 1430 and 1930.

Jen's bowel movements have suddenly changed over the last two months to three to five times a day and mostly watery. This makes her sister very anxious about taking her out of the house. Despite not losing weight over the last two months, she hasn't gained any weight either, which concerns her sister as well.

Write out a few potentials of what you think could be causing this sudden bowel movement change.

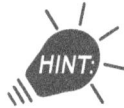

> **HINT:**
>
> Explore any recent activity or medication changes, or any bouts of acute illness that may have changed her digestive systems nutrient and water absorption capacity.

Commentary

Here are some potential causes of Jen's bowel movement changes to investigate further.

1. **Medication changes:**

   Has Jen started on any new medications or had a change in medication dosage in the last two months? Before making any dietary changes, explore whether the observed change in bowel habits may be attributed to any change in her usual medications. Several medications, especially antibiotics,[1] are infamous for affecting bowel habits, therefore it's important to explore this potential in detail by asking specific questions about medication dose and timing changes that may have taken place. If recent antibiotic use is confirmed, a period of probiotics may be warranted to rebuild the gut microbiome.[2]

2. **Gastrointestinal infection:**

   An underlying infection, such as of clostridium difficile, could be causing the sudden onset of frequent and watery stools. A stool sample to explore this cause may be warranted and can be broached with her primary doctor. Post-infectious irritable bowel syndrome (IBS) may also be plausible after a period of gut infection.[3] In this case, she may benefit from switching to a lower fermentable oligosaccharides, disaccharides, monosaccharides and polyols (FODMAP)-containing formula.

3. **Malabsorption on the background of acute illness:**
    Has Jen recently been on a course of antibiotics or had a hospital admission which may have affected her gut microbiome and nutrient absorption capacity? Jen might not be absorbing fat and fat-soluble nutrients properly, leading to watery stools and an inability to gain weight. What colour are her watery bowel motions? If her stools are yellow in colour, this may be indicative of fat malabsorption (i.e. steatorrhea). Black coloured stools may mean an upper gastrointestinal tract bleed such as a stomach ulcer perforation. Bright red blood may mean bleeding in the large intestine or rectum, such as in the case of haemorrhoids. It's warranted to liaise with Jen's primary doctor to comprehensively assess her stool composition and colour. [4]

4. **Fibre inadequacy:**
    Is Jen on a fibre-containing formula? Given the sudden onset of her diarrhoea, Jen's symptoms are unlikely to be formula related as she had been on that formula prior to the stool changes. Nonetheless, fibre in the enteral formula is indisputably important. One should be aiming for at least 25 grams (g) of fibre per day, with the dose dispersed across the day. If Jen isn't on a fibre-containing formula, it would be ideal to consider introducing this into her feeding regimen at 25% of the target dose and titrating up accordingly over a few days/weeks depending on tolerance until target is reached.[5]

5. **Diarrhoea overflow:**

    Loose stools aren't always loose stools. This may be related to chronic constipation with resultant overflow.[6] An abdominal examination, ultrasound or x-ray conducted or ordered by her primary doctor could support investigating underlying chronic constipation. If overflow diarrhoea is the cause, medical management followed by longer term optimisation of fibre, fluid, mobility and regular aperients may be considered.

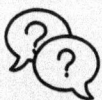

Post-case reflective questions

▶ How would you prioritise investigating potential causes of Jen's bowel movement changes (e.g. medication, diet, hydration)?

▶ How would you modify Jen's nutrition plan to address the watery stools without compromising her weight maintenance goals?

Notes

1. Ramirez J, Guarner F, Bustos Fernandez L, Maruy A, Sdepanian VL and Cohen H (2020) 'Antibiotics as Major Disruptors of Gut Microbiota'. *Frontiers in Cellular and Infection Microbiology*, 10(10). doi:https://doi.org/10.3389/fcimb.2020.572912. Available at: https://pubmed.ncbi.nlm.nih.gov/33330122/#:~:text=Antibiotic%20use%20can%20have%20several,and%20recurrent%20Clostridioides%20difficile%20infections.

2. Newberry SJ (2012) 'Probiotics for the Prevention and Treatment of Antibiotic-Associated Diarrhea'. *JAMA*, [online] 307(18), p.1959. doi:https://doi.org/10.1001/jama.2012.3507. Available at: https://pubmed.ncbi.nlm.nih.gov/22570464/

3. Lupu VV, Ghiciuc CM, Stefanescu G, Mihai CM, Popp A, Sasaran MO, Bozomitu L, Starcea IM, Adam Raileanu A and Lupu A (2023) 'Emerging role of the gut microbiome in post-infectious irritable bowel syndrome: A literature review'. *World J Gastroenterol*. 2023 Jun 7;29(21):3241-3256. doi: 10.3748/wjg.v29.i21.3241. PMID: 37377581; PMCID: PMC10292139. Available at: https://www.ncbi.nlm.nih.gov/pmc/articles/PMC10292139/

4. Mayo Clinic (n.d.) *Stool color: When to worry.* [online] Available at: https://www.mayoclinic.org/stool-color/expert-answers/faq-20058080#:~:text=Stool%20comes%20in%20a%20range

5. So D, Gibson PR, Muir JG and Yao CK (2021) 'Dietary fibres and IBS: translating functional characteristics to clinical value in the era of personalised medicine'. *Gut.* [online] doi:https://doi.org/10.1136/gutjnl-2021-324891. Available at: https://pubmed.ncbi.nlm.nih.gov/34417199/

6. Arasaradnam RP, Brown S, Forbes A, Fox MR, Hungin P, Kelman L, Major G, O'Connor M, Sanders DS, Sinha R, Smith SC, Thomas P and Walters JRF (2018) 'Guidelines for the investigation of chronic diarrhoea in adults: British Society of Gastroenterology', 3rd edition. *Gut.* [online] 67(8), pp.1380–1399. doi:https://doi.org/10.1136/gutjnl-2017-315909. Available at: https://www.ncbi.nlm.nih.gov/pmc/articles/PMC6204957/

Raquel –
Overnight
Watery Stools

Raquel is a 37-year-old woman with cerebral palsy who does not have the ability to verbally communicate, move the right side of her body or swallow food. Raquel lives with her foster parents and brings them immense joy. Her bubbly personality and radiant smile make her a beacon of happiness wherever she goes.

Raquel has a percutaneous endoscopic gastrostomy (PEG), size 20 Fr, skin disc positioned at 3.5 cm at skin level and secured with a balloon inflated with 7 ml of water.

Her feeding regimen consists of a 1.5 kcal/ml fibre-containing formula at 90 ml/hour (hr) from 2100 to 0800 (11 hours via electric pump), and 125 ml of a 1.2 kcal/ml formula administered as a syringe bolus feed via gravity at 1400. Additionally, she receives 175 ml of water every two hours during the day and medications at 0800 and 2000.

Her foster parents are concerned about her bowel output, which is highest overnight and consists of watery stools that often cause skin irritation if not cleaned up immediately (understandably difficult to do at 0400!). To address this, a trial of switching Raquel to daytime feeds in a bolus fashion to mimic normal eating patterns is considered.

What do you need to consider to aid with this transition?

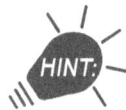

> **HINT:**
>
> Start by writing out key questions to determine Raquel's daily routine to aid in understanding what a daytime bolus regimen could potentially look like for her and her foster parents.

Commentary

When considering Raquel's transition from receiving her nutrition overnight via electric pump to during the day via syringe bolus gravity, there are two potential approaches:

1. Cold turkey
2. Gradual

Considerations to determine best approach

To make an informed decision about which approach to take, consider the following questions:

▶ Has Raquel experienced unintentional, undesirable weight loss in the last six months? Understanding this aspect of her nutritional status is crucial to assess the fragility of her body and the potential impact of missing out on essential calorie provision during a transition from overnight to daytime nutrition.

▶ Has Raquel had any hospital admissions in the last six months? If so, a more gradual approach may be advisable to avoid compromising nutritional intake during the recovery period following an acute hospital admission.

▶ What is Raquel's daily routine like in terms of awake times, sleep times and overall lifestyle? Understanding her daily activities and schedule can help tailor the feeding plan to fit seamlessly into her life (and that of her foster parents).

▶ Is Raquel able to communicate any discomfort or preferences during mealtimes? Ensuring her comfort and addressing any preferences she may have can enhance the overall success of the transition. An example of this is whether she is able to move her eyes to indicate "yes" or "no" when asked about feelings of fullness or bloating during a syringe bolus feed, which would usually be a larger volume of nutrition provision in a shorter time frame than electric pump feeds.

▶ What is Raquel's maximum bolus tolerance rate? This will help you determine how many boluses a day she'll need if, for example, she needs 800 ml of a 2.0 kcal/ml formula (i.e. 200 ml bolus four times a day or 133 ml bolus six times a day). Any history of gastrointestinal surgery or resections in Raquel's medical background may potentially give some clues around her capacity to tolerate larger volume boluses. For example, if Raquel has undergone a gastric sleeve, the amount of formula she can tolerate in a single bolus feed may be affected.[1]

▶ Does Raquel have insulin-dependent diabetes? If yes, a gradual approach may be safest. Additionally, close collaboration with her endocrinologist is essential for the transition to bolus daytime feeding, including adjustments to the timing and dosages of long- and short-acting insulin medications. Refer to Case 14 for further exploration of insulin-dependent diabetes and tube feeding.

► Is Raquel taking any medication during the day that requires an empty stomach, such as Parkinson's disease medication or a particular antibiotic? This would affect the timings of the daytime boluses.

► Is there a support system in place at home for the transition? Does she have all the equipment needed to implement this new regimen? Do her foster parents need training on how to administer a syringe bolus mealtime via gravity?

► Does her formula need to be changed to a more concentrated formulation like a 2.0 kcal/ml or a bolus-friendly packaging amount like a 125 ml or 200 ml bottle rather than a 1000 ml bottle that would require refrigeration between boluses? How soon can this new formula be trialled to ensure tolerance?

► Refer to Case 1 for consideration of loose stools which may still need to be considered for Raquel.

Example of a cold turkey approach

Cold turkey may mean switching to a 2.0 kcal/ml formula and commencing feeds from dinner time (~1800) to bedtime (~2100), then commencing the next day with a feeding regimen of 200 ml formula bolus at 0800, 1200, 1600 and 2000 (totalling 800 ml formula in a 24-hour period, assuming this is the amount she requires for adequate macronutrient and micronutrient intake).

Example of a gradual approach

Gradual may mean reducing the overnight feeding calorie provision by 500 calories and then providing that amount as an additional mealtime or bolus the next day. This approach would then be used for the remainder of the week until all calorie intake has been swapped over. Bear in mind Raquel is on a 1.5 kcal/ml formula, so for this approach, switching her over to a 2 kcal/ml formula first may be warranted in order to require less volume of formula in a bolus.

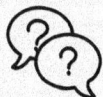

Post-case reflective questions

▶ How would you structure a new feeding plan for Raquel to fit her daytime routine without disrupting her foster parents' caregiving schedule?

▶ What are potential risks in shifting from overnight to daytime feeds? How would you mitigate them?

▶ How would you involve Raquel's foster parents in the decision-making process to ensure the new plan is feasible?

Notes

1. Kim TH, Lee YJ, Bae K, Park JH, Hong SC, Jung EJ, Ju YT, Jeong CY, Park TJ, Park M, Kim JE and Jeong SH (2019) 'The investigation of diet recovery after distal gastrectomy'. *Medicine* (Baltimore). 98(41):e17543. doi: 10.1097/MD.0000000000017543. PMID: 31593134; PMCID: PMC6799850. Available at: https://www.ncbi.nlm.nih.gov/pmc/articles/PMC6799850/#:~:text=Six%20months%20after%20gastrectomy%2C%20half,at%20the%201st%20POM%20(Fig

Case 3

Geoff –
Continuous
to Bolus

At 50 years old, Geoff had a stroke which has affected his speech and swallowing but definitely does not define him. What truly defines Geoff is his immense heart, his gentle and kind soul, and the boundless joy he brings to his family and friends.

Geoff uses a low-profile gastrostomy tube (also can be referred to as a 'button tube'), which is 24 Fr in size with a shaft length of 3.5 cm. He lives at home with his loving younger brother.

Geoff's current feeding regimen is 100 ml/hr of a 1.0 kcal/ml formula delivered continuously for 24 hours a day from a 1000 ml ready-to-hang bottle. His brother stops and starts the feeds regularly throughout the day to accommodate activities like showering, hydrotherapy and other engagements. Geoff's brother would love for him to be on a feeding plan that better accommodates his daily activities, but he is concerned because when Geoff first had his stroke the hospital advised him that Geoff could only tolerate 100 ml/hr of formula and must remain on the electric pump.

How would you go about this?

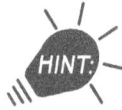

> **HINT:**
>
> Transitioning Geoff to a more suitable feeding plan involves collaborative steps with his brother to ease his concerns, including discussing a higher concentration formula and assessing gastrointestinal function.

Commentary

Transitioning Geoff to a feeding plan that better accommodates his daily activities requires careful consideration and collaboration.

Transition steps to consider

Step 1: Discussion with brother

► Hospital contact: Identify any communication from the hospital from Geoff's last admission (if within a reasonable time frame) to understand the recommendations given around maximum feed rate and delivery method.

► Daily routine: Learn about Geoff's daily routine, activities and specific challenges in managing his current feeding schedule. This will help you determine how flexible the feeding regime needs to be based on Geoff's activities.

► Benefits explanation: Discuss the benefits of bolus feeding, including its positive impact on muscle mass maintenance, blood glucose levels, bowel function, sleep quality and overall quality of life for Geoff. It has been reported as the more common home tube feeding delivery method.[1]

► Communication and monitoring: Determine if Geoff can communicate symptoms like bloating or pain, and discuss how this can assist in monitoring his feed tolerance.

- Delivery preferences: Evaluate whether they prefer to use an electric pump for convenience and ease of set-up, or due to fear of intolerance to other delivery methods such as syringe bolus gravity or gravity drip feeding. Understanding this will help your counsel accordingly.

- New formula consideration: Assess their comfort level with trying a new formula, such as a 2 kcal/ml formulation, which would reduce Geoff's daily requirement of formula volume by half (i.e. 1200 ml versus 2400 ml).

Step 2: Change to a higher concentration formula

- Start by changing one aspect at a time, such as introducing a higher concentration formula first.

- As a first step, consider continuing 24-hour feeds using a pump but at 50 ml/hr with a 2.0 kcal/ml formula to see how Geoff tolerates the formula. A higher concentration formula would simplify the transition to a bolus feeding regimen in the long run as the volume of boluses required would be half the volume of his current formula.

Step 3: Assess gastrointestinal function

- If the concerns around Geoff's maximum feed tolerance rate being 100 ml/hr limit the potential to creatively flex his feeding plan, check if Geoff has had a recent gastric emptying study or if his primary doctor thinks it would be warranted to check gastric motility.

- Work with Geoff's primary doctor to understand how to optimise his gastrointestinal function with further investigations or medications to improve motility should it be an issue.

Step 4: Training and education

▶ Provide training for Geoff's brother on transitioning to a bolus daytime feeding regimen, including correct feeding positions, bolus feeding using a 60ml syringe or an electric pump, and recognising signs of intolerance.

Step 5: Hydration and medication management

▶ Transitioning to a more concentrated formula means less overall fluid provided. Any fluid deficit can be met by increasing water flushes to maintain hydration.

▶ Review and align Geoff's medication schedule with the daytime bolus feed times to minimise frequent handling of the feeding tube. This will need collaboration with his primary doctor.

Step 6: Monitor and follow-up

▶ Change the feeding regimen on a Monday so that healthcare providers are available throughout the week for troubleshooting.

▶ Schedule a follow-up appointment two to three days into the new regimen to monitor for any signs of intolerance (e.g. bloating, abdomen distension, vomiting, diarrhoea).[2]

Step 7: Support services

▶ Connect Geoff's brother with home nursing support to assist with the transition.

▶ Ensure his primary doctor is aware of the transition and available for support.

Step 8: Empower autonomy

▶ Encourage flexibility in the feeding regimen. Every day does not need to look exactly like the one before in terms of mealtimes and even delivery method. Things can and should evolve with each day's activities.

▶ Emphasise that, like oral eaters, it's normal to vary the feeding schedule and volumes.

Step 9: Documentation and communication

▶ Document the full transition feeding regimen and walk Geoff's brother through it step by step. Remember he is likely to be very nervous about the change, and without constant monitoring of a hospital setting, you'll need to be available for phone support.

▶ Maintain open communication channels for any questions or concerns during the transition period.

Example transition regimen

Week 1 – Transition regimen

Day 1: Change to a 2.0 kcal/ml formula and run at 50 ml/hr continuously (24 hrs).

Day 2: Cease the feeding at 2000.

Day 3: Increase the feed rate to 100 ml/hr and run for 12 hours from 0800 to 2000.

Day 4: Bolus his mealtimes as follows:

- 100 ml/hr from 0800 to 1200
- 100 ml/hr from 1400 to 1800
- 100 ml/hr from 2000 to 0000

Total formula provision in 24 hours = 1200 ml.

Week 2 – Reach target feeding regimen

Day 1: Bolus his mealtimes as follows:

- 135 ml/hr from 0800 to 1100
- 135 ml/hr from 1400 to 1700
- 135 ml/hr from 2000 to 2300

Total formula provision in 24 hours = 1215 ml.

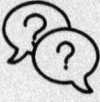

Post-case reflective questions

- How would you build Geoff's brother's confidence in transitioning from continuous to bolus feeding?
- What would be your approach if Geoff were unable to tolerate higher feed concentrations?
- How could you support Geoff's daily activities while ensuring he continues to meet his nutritional needs?

Notes

1. Hubbard GP, Andrews S, White S, Simpson G, Topen S, Carnie L, Murphy C, Collins R, Davies J, Owen A, Barker J, Green L, Patel I, Ridgway J, Lenchner J, Faerber J, Pearce L, Meanwell H, Kominek N and Stark L (2019) 'A survey of bolus tube feeding prevalence and practice in adult patients requiring home enteral tube feeding'. *British Journal of Nutrition*, 122(11), pp.1271–1278. doi:https://doi.org/10.1017/s000711451900223x. Available at: https://pubmed.ncbi.nlm.nih.gov/31782379

2. Jenkins B, Calder PC and Marino LV (2022) 'A systematic review of the definitions and prevalence of feeding intolerance in critically ill adults'. *Clinical Nutrition ESPEN*, 49, 92–102. https://doi.org/10.1016/j.clnesp.2022.04.014. Available at: https://clinicalnutritionespen.com/article/S2405-4577(22)00239-X/abstract

Sarah –
A Gaseous
Problem

Sarah, a 27-year-old, shares an unbreakable bond with her father, Larry. They're not just father and daughter; they're the closest of friends. Their connection is unmatched in its sincerity and affection. Despite Sarah's lifelong challenges following an acquired brain injury, her spirit remains vibrant and unique.

Sarah relies entirely on a PEG tube for her nutritional needs. Her current regimen involves 240 g of a 1.5 kcal/ml formula mixed with 1000 ml of water, which is prepared by Larry every morning and stored in the fridge. Sarah receives three bolus feeds per day of 270 ml of formula, with 30 ml of water before, 60 ml after and an additional 250 ml of water midmorning. The formula is decanted into an empty container for each bolus and administered as a gravity drip feed.[1]

Larry reports that Sarah has always had a problem with wind and moans in pain regularly throughout the day, especially around mealtimes, and also during the night, 1–2 times after midnight.

What are some potential solutions to trial for her wind problem?

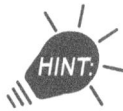

> **HINT:**
>
> Consider air ingestion, constipation and feed delivery method as potential factors contributing to Sarah's wind issue.

Commentary

Here are some potential solutions to trial:

1. **Switch to liquid formula:**
   The practice of mixing powder formula in water each morning may introduce air bubbles in the formula mixture, potentially contributing to the reported gas build-up and wind pain experienced by Sarah. This aspect of formula preparation warrants attention; perhaps switching to a liquid commercial formula may be a worthwhile trial as a first option to minimise air ingestion.

2. **Explore her feeding position:**
   Sarah should ideally be sitting upright during mealtimes. A comprehensive review of her wheelchair and seating position should be considered. Check when her last formal wheelchair assessment by an occupational therapist was conducted, and encourage Larry to arrange a follow-up. Optimising aspects of her wheelchair configuration may enhance her positioning, body posture and thus stomach capacity during mealtimes.

3. **Investigate her gastric motility:**
   Diagnostic investigations carried out by her primary doctor might be necessary to check for gastroparesis or gastroesophageal reflux disease (GORD).[2] If diagnosed, these conditions can be managed with medications to

improve food movement through her digestive system and alleviate gas build-up.

4. **Vent her stomach regularly:**
   Introduce a proactive stomach venting plan, venting her stomach approximately 15 minutes before each bolus feed to release accumulated gas, potentially reducing Sarah's discomfort. A nurse experienced in feeding tubes can teach Larry how to vent properly and what precautions to take.[3]

5. **Assess her current bowel habits (i.e. stool output):**
   Conduct a thorough assessment of Sarah's bowel activity to understand her gastrointestinal motility better. Evaluate the efficacy of her current bowel regimen, including fibre content in her formula, fluid intake, and laxative medication dosage and timing (if applicable to her). Involve her primary doctor in this review and consider adjustments such as introducing aperients, enemas or suppositories to alleviate digestive system pressure.

6. **Review fibre and FODMAP content of the formula:**
   The majority of enteral formulas are considered low lactose and low FODMAP, however this depends on the fibre composition. A more gel or bulking type fibre rather than fermentable (gas-producing) fibre may be better suited to Sarah.[4]

7. **Advocate for a PEG-Jejunostomy (PEG-J) insertion :**
   In some cases of severe gas build up, abdominal distension and discomfort, liaising with a doctor regarding the appropriateness of a PEG-J tube may be warranted. Such tubes would have two ports – one going to the stomach and one to the jejunum. This would allow the gastric port to be used for decompression, draining out fluids and air to control pressure build up, while the jejunal port provides feeding access. Draining from the gastric port can occur periodically or around mealtimes to relieve pressure from fluid build-up, or it can be set to "free drain" for certain periods, either day or night. This method may lead to extra fluid and electrolyte losses though, requiring close coordination with a doctor.[5]

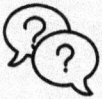

Post-case reflective questions

- ▶ How would you determine whether Sarah's wind problem is related to her feeding position or formula preparation?
- ▶ What alternative methods could be trialled to relieve her gas symptoms?
- ▶ How would you collaborate with Sarah's father to optimise her comfort during and after meals?

Notes

1. Ichimaru S (2018) 'Methods of Enteral Nutrition Administration in Critically Ill Patients: Continuous, Cyclic, Intermittent, and Bolus Feeding'. *Nutrition in Clinical Practice*, 33(6), 790–795. https://doi. org/10.1002/ncp.10105. Available at: https://pubmed.ncbi.nlm.nih. gov/29924423/

2. Banks KP, Syed K, Parekh M and McWhorter N (2023) *Gastric Emptying Scan*. [online] Available at: https://www.ncbi.nlm.nih.gov/books/ NBK531503/

3. Rajan A, Wangrattanapranee P, Kessler J, Kidambi TD and Tabibian JH (2022, April 27) 'Gastrostomy tubes: Fundamentals, periprocedural considerations, and best practices'. *World J Gastrointest Surg.* 14(4):286-303. doi: 10.4240/wjgs.v14.i4.286. PMID: 35664365; PMCID: PMC9131834. Available at: https://www.ncbi.nlm.nih.gov/pmc/articles/ PMC9131834/

4. Halmos EP (2013) 'Role of FODMAP content in enteral nutrition-associated diarrhea'. *Journal of Gastroenterology and Hepatology*, 28, 25–28. https://doi.org/10.1111/jgh.12272. Available at: https://onlinelibrary. wiley.com/doi/10.1111/jgh.12272

5. Ohkubo H, Fuyuki A, Arimoto J, Higurashi T, Nonaka T, Inoh Y, Iida H, Inamori M, Kaneda T, Nakajima A. Efficacy of percutaneous endoscopic gastro-jejunostomy (PEG-J) decompression therapy for patients with chronic intestinal pseudo-obstruction (CIPO). Neurogastroenterol Motil. 2017 Dec;29(12). doi: 10.1111/nmo.13127. Epub 2017 Jun 20. PMID: 28631871. Available at: https://pubmed.ncbi.nlm.nih.gov/28631871/

Anatoli –
Tube Weaning

Anatoli, 59 years old, is praised by his wife for his intelligence and wit. He recently had a subtotal gastrectomy and revision of his gastric bypass surgery. A jejunostomy (JEJ), as a 16 Fr tube, was inserted during the surgery.

He was discharged from hospital meeting all his nutritional needs through the feeding tube with the following regimen: 80 ml/hr of a 1.5 kcal/ml formula from 1700 to 0900 (16 hours), plus 80 ml water flushes before and after. This provides him with 1400 ml of fluid and 76 g of protein daily.

Anatoli's surgeon advised that he can have clear fluids for the next week through his mouth, then gradually progress to free fluids and eventually eat a soft diet based on his tolerance.

What strategy could you recommend to help him wean off his feeding tube?

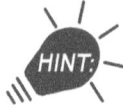

HINT:

Consider a strategy that combines maximising his oral intake with gradual adjustments to his tube feeding regimen based on his meal consumption.

Commentary

By adopting a 'food first' approach and tailoring tube feeds based on his oral intake, Anatoli can gradually transition off the feeding tube. Let's explore these strategies in more detail:

Food first approach

► **Maximise oral intake:**

- Fortify foods: Enrich meals with protein powder, milk powder or other high-calorie ingredients to increase protein and calorie intake without significantly increasing the volume of food needing to be consumed.

- Nutrient-rich snacks: Introduce high-calorie, high-protein snacks between meals to boost overall intake and reduce reliance on tube feeds.

- Regular meals: Encourage small, frequent meals (5–6 times a day) to make eating more manageable and to stimulate appetite.

► **Use oral nutritional supplements (ONS):**

- Supplemental drinks: Use commercially made or homemade high-calorie shakes to increase calorie and protein intake orally.

- Strategic timing: Consume ONS between meals to avoid reducing appetite for main meals and to ensure additional nutritional support.

Micronutrient supplementation

▶ Given Anatoli's surgical history of a gastric bypass followed by a subtotal gastrectomy, it is crucial to ensure he receives adequate micronutrient intake. The most common deficiencies after gastric bypass include thiamine, vitamin B12, vitamin D, iron and copper.[1]

▶ Close collaboration with Anatoli's surgeon and primary doctor is essential to optimise the supplementation of these nutrients.

Tailor tube feeds based on oral intake

▶ If partial meal consumption: If Anatoli consumes half of an oral meal, follow it up with 80 ml/hr of formula running for two hours via pump or administer 160 ml through a syringe, gravity assisted, into the feeding tube. Close collaboration with the surgeon is key when making such changes.

▶ If full meal consumption: Omit the tube feed if the entire meal is consumed. This encourages increased oral intake while ensuring nutritional needs are met.

▶ Shift tube feeding to overnight to avoid potential disruption of daytime oral intake opportunities. For example, commence the tube feeding at 80 ml/hr from 2200 to 0800 (8 hours). This provides approximately half of his nutritional requirements overnight, allowing for more focus on oral intake during the day. Anatoli would then reduce the number of hours he receives the overnight nutrition based on his oral intake throughout the day. If there are concerns regarding the maximum pump rate for jejunal feeding or the amount of formula administered via syringe through Anatoli's JEJ, please refer to Case 19 for further discussion on this.

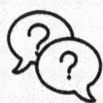

💬 Post-case reflective questions

► What factors would influence your decision to adjust Anatoli's feeding regimen as he transitions to oral intake?

► How would you monitor his progress to ensure adequate nutrition as his tube feeding is reduced?

► What role does Anatoli's wife play in ensuring a successful weaning process, and how can you support her?

Notes

1. Saltzman E and Karl JP (2013) 'Nutrient deficiencies after gastric bypass surgery'. *Annual Review of Nutrition*, [online] 33, pp.183–203. doi:https://doi.org/10.1146/annurev-nutr-071812-161225. Available at: https://pubmed.ncbi.nlm.nih.gov/23642197/#:~:text=The%20most%20common%20clinically%20relevant,D%2C%20iron%2C%20and%20copper

Aiden – Tube Assessment and Blockage

Aiden, a 21-year-old young man, was born with microcephaly and was later diagnosed with cerebral palsy. Everyday tasks like moving and eating have become more and more challenging for him over the years. But it doesn't hold him back from enjoying his favourite music: heavy metal.

He is unable to take in enough nutrition by mouth and, as a result, is dependent on a PEG feeding tube.

During your initial assessment, you notice he doesn't have a medical or nursing professional overseeing his feeding tube and stoma site care. To arrange for this necessary support for Aiden, what details could you collect during your assessment about the feeding tube itself to facilitate a detailed referral to the appropriate health professional?

The following week you receive a call from Aiden's carer that it appears the tube is blocked. What advice would you give over the phone to help them attempt to unblock the tube?

Lina Breik

Commentary

Feeding tube details

During your assessment, it's essential to gather feeding tube details, including:

1. Date of initial insertion
2. Date of the last tube change
3. Date of next routine tube change
4. Brand of the tube, specifying the manufacturing company
5. Type of tube (e.g. PEG, PEJ, RIG, low-profile gastrostomy or jejunostomy, JEJ)
6. Tube size, indicated in French (Fr)
7. Whether the tube is ENFit-ended or not. ENFit is a standardised connector for enteral feeding tubes that prevents misconnections and improves individual safety by ensuring compatibility only with equipment designed for administering into the digestive system, as opposed to intravenously (i.e. to the blood)[1]
8. Insertion method: endoscope, radiology or surgery
9. Termination point: stomach or small intestine (i.e. duodenum or jejunum?)
10. Anchoring device and tube removal method:
    a. Anchoring device: balloon, rigid flange, collapsible flange, other
    b. Removal: traction, endoscope or surgery

11. Number of ports on the tube

12. Level at the top of the skin disc (the skin disc may also be referred to as an external flange)

13. Condition of the tube itself (i.e. any discolouration, kinks or cracks)

14. Condition of the stoma site, considering factors such as pain, redness, itchiness, heat, colour of discharge (if any) and details about their daily care routine

Feeding tube blockage

It is important to ensure all individuals who have feeding tubes at home have a documented emergency plan specifying who to call in the event of a mishap such as the tube being blocked or dislodging. However, assuming this plan is not available for Aiden, here are some steps you may advise over the phone:[2]

1. **Push-pull technique:**
   Instruct Aiden's carer to attempt flushing the tube with warm water using a syringe. Gently push and pull the plunger to create a gentle flow. Sometimes a smaller syringe (e.g. 10 ml rather than standard 60 ml) can help, as it provides a different level of pressure.

2. **Check for kinks or bends:**
   Ask Aiden's carer to inspect the external portion of the tube for any kinks or bends that might be obstructing the flow. Straightening the tube carefully can sometimes resolve the issue.

3. **External massage:**
   Gently massage the external part of the tube between the thumb and fingers to dislodge any material stuck inside.

4. **Soaking the connector port:**
   If the blockage is suspected in the connector port, soak it in warm water, especially for tubes with a removable port. This can be done while the tube is still attached to the patient, with the tube cap open for soaking.

If the blockage persists, the decision-making juncture involves either waiting until the next business day to consult with his specialist or primary doctor for tube replacement, or proceeding to his local emergency department (ED). Which road to take depends on several factors. For example, if there are any time-sensitive medications potentially putting him at risk of not being able to ingest them if the feeding tube remains blocked, it would be warranted to advise Aiden to head to his local ED (taking a spare feeding tube with him).

Prevention of feeding tube blockages

Steps to avoid such a mishap from happening again:

▶ Ensure frequent water flushes in his daily routine. This would include water before and after all boluses or continuous administration, as well as between mealtimes as appropriate for his lifestyle.

▶ Ensure correct medication administration, inclusive of:

- crushing and administering tablets one by one
- using water flushes between each medication administration
- opting for liquid medications where available.

▶ Ensure his carers are trained in correct medication administration and nutrition provision through a feeding tube.

▶ Ensure Aiden has a spare feeding tube or two at home for future emergencies.

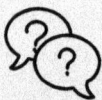

Post-case reflective questions

▶ How would you ensure that Aiden's carers are adequately trained to prevent future tube blockages?

▶ What proactive measures would you take to maintain the long-term functionality of Aiden's PEG tube?

Notes

1. Global Engineered Device Supplier Association (n.d.) *ENFit*®. [online] Stay Connected® by GEDSA™. Available at: https://stayconnected.org/enfit/ [Accessed 18 Sep. 2024]

2. Agency for Clinical Innovation (2015, March) *A Clinician's Guide: Caring for people with gastrostomy tubes and devices – From pre-insertion to ongoing care and removal.* Available at: https://aci.health.nsw.gov.au/__data/ assets/pdf_file/0017/251063/ACI-Clinicians-guide-caring-people-gastrostomy-tubes-devices.pdf

Aiden – Tube Dislodgement

Aiden's carer calls you frantically on a Monday afternoon and states that he has tugged at his PEG tube and that "more of the tube is dangling down from his stomach hole than it was the day before".

What would you advise the carer to do in this instance?

Commentary

Immediate actions

1. Refrain from feeding, administering medication, or providing water through the tube.

2. Given in Aiden's case the tube is still in the stoma (i.e. the surgically formed hole through which the feeding tube enters the body), avoid any sudden movements that may make the tube fall completely out, and call the health professional overseeing his feeding tube management for advice around next steps. Granted he isn't on any time-sensitive medications, it may be OK for Aiden to present to his doctors' clinic the next business day knowing he will miss some nutrition until then. The stoma hole begins to close anytime between 8 and 24 hours of the tube falling out of the body, hence the importance of avoiding any sudden movements in Aiden's case.[1]

3. If the tube had completely fallen out of Aiden's body, contact the health professional responsible for his feeding tube as soon as possible. They may advise his carer to reinsert the tube back into the stoma gently and tape it to his abdomen, preventing the hole from closing.

4. In case time-sensitive medication through the tube is necessary or if attempts to contact the specified health professional are unsuccessful, Aiden should proceed to the nearest ED with his spare tube in hand.

Long-term considerations for dislodgement prevention

▶ Consider the use of an abdominal binder or gastrostomy belt to tuck the PEG tube away so as to minimise the chance of accidental dislodgement.

▶ If Aiden frequently pulls at the PEG, and therefore dislodgement is likely to happen again, consider liaising with his primary doctor about transitioning him to a low-profile gastrostomy tube (a.k.a. a 'button').

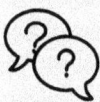

Post-case reflective questions

▶ What instructions would you give Aiden's carer to prevent tube dislodgement in the future?

▶ How would you ensure that Aiden's carers have the confidence and tools to manage a potential tube dislodgement emergency?

▶ What factors would you consider when deciding whether Aiden would truly benefit from a low-profile gastrostomy tube, and what changes does this type of tube come with from an equipment perspective?

Notes

1. Agency for Clinical Innovation (2015, March) *A Clinician's Guide: Caring for people with gastrostomy tubes and devices – From pre-insertion to ongoing care and removal.* Available at: https://aci.health.nsw.gov.au/__data/ assets/pdf_file/0017/251063/ACI-Clinicians-guide-caring-people-gastrostomy-tubes-devices.pdf

Tahir – Gastric Fluid Leak

Tahir is a resilient and determined 68-year-old gentleman who has faced the challenges of life head-on. Several months ago, he underwent a gastrostomy tube placement following a left-sided brain stroke that diminished his swallowing capacity. Despite this setback, Tahir maintains a positive outlook on life and approaches each day with courage and grace.

His decision to choose a low-profile gastrostomy tube (22 Fr, shaft length of 2.7cm, and anchored in place by a balloon inflated with 7 ml of water) was driven by the goal of enhancing his comfort with the least visible tube option available. Tahir meets 100% of his nutrition and hydration needs through his feeding tube.

During your recent assessment of Tahir's nutrition, you notice gastric fluid leaking from his stoma site. What are some potential causes and solutions for this leakage?

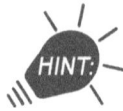

> **HINT:**
>
> Consider exploring tube placement, balloon inflation, stoma integrity and gastric motility.

Lina Breik

Commentary

Potential causes[1]

1. **Balloon is not inflated enough:**
   If the balloon anchoring the feeding tube in place from the inside is deflated, it may not provide an adequate seal at the stoma site. This can result in leakage around the tube and reduced stability.

2. **Balloon rupture:**
   A ruptured balloon will fail to keep the feeding tube properly anchored. This can cause the tube to move, leading to leakage and potential displacement.

3. **Gastrostomy tube position:**
   If the gastrostomy tube is improperly positioned, it can affect the efficiency of feeding and cause discomfort or leakage.

4. **An ill-fitting device:**
   If Tahir has recently had any significant weight gain or loss, particularly around his abdominal area, the current shaft length of his tube may not be the best fit for him. This could lead to leakage around the site.

5. **Poor gastric emptying:**
   Slow gastric emptying or gastroparesis can cause a build-up of gastric contents, leading to increased pressure and potential leakage around the feeding tube.

Potential solutions[1]

1. **Escalate to the doctor or nurse overseeing his feeding tube and stoma site care:**
   It is essential to escalate to the right healthcare professionals who can assess the situation thoroughly. They may decide to replace the feeding tube or inflate the anchoring balloon with a higher volume to improve the stoma seal. Tahir may even be taught to check the balloon volume himself at home on a regular basis, if deemed appropriate, to prevent such a mishap.

2. **Relieve any constipation Tahir may be experiencing:**
   Addressing constipation can reduce abdominal pressure, which in turn can alleviate some of the stress on the stomach and the stoma site. This may involve increasing fluid intake and dietary fibre or using laxatives under guidance from his primary doctor.

3. **Venting the gastric contents out of the feeding tube between mealtimes:**
   By venting the tube away from mealtimes, excess gas and gastric contents can be released, reducing pressure within the stomach. This can help prevent discomfort and

leakage, especially if done regularly between feeds. Tahir can be taught to vent his tube by a doctor or nurse.

4. **Regular prokinetics after medical review:**
Prokinetic medications can enhance gastric motility, helping to empty the stomach more efficiently.[2] After assessing Tahir, his primary doctor may prescribe such medications, which would reduce the risk of pressure build-up and associated complications. It may also be appropriate to also consider some barrier cream to protect the stoma site skin. A doctor or nurse can advise on the best option for Tahir.

5. **Review the nutrition regimen:**
Re-evaluating Tahir's feeding regimen might be necessary after the previous solutions have been addressed. Reducing the volume of each bolus feed or mealtime, or transitioning from bolus to continuous feeding, can decrease the pressure on the stomach and stoma site.

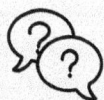

Post-case reflective questions

► What do you think is within scope of practice for a dietitian to advise in such a situation?

► How would you educate Tahir about preventing future leaks, especially regarding balloon inflation and stoma care?

Notes

1. Agency for Clinical Innovation (2015, March) *A Clinician's Guide: Caring for people with gastrostomy tubes and devices – From pre-insertion to ongoing care and removal.* Available at: https://aci.health.nsw.gov.au/__data/assets/pdf_file/0017/251063/ACI-Clinicians-guide-caring-people-gastrostomy-tubes-devices.pdf

2. Camilleri M and Atieh J (2021) 'New Developments in Prokinetic Therapy for Gastric Motility Disorders'. *Frontiers in Pharmacology*, 12, 711500. https://doi.org/10.3389/fphar.2021.711500. Available at: https://www.ncbi.nlm.nih.gov/pmc/articles/PMC8421525/

Amina – Progressive Weight Gain

Amina, a 26-year-old female, requires long-term enteral feeding after a life-changing event that resulted in a traumatic brain injury (TBI) about a year ago. Despite her daily challenges, she finds joy in the simple pleasures of life, whether it's watching movies or connecting with loved ones.

She has an 18 Fr PEG tube and has experienced a weight gain of 15.4 kg in the last six months, posing increased challenges for her caregivers in terms of mobility and hygiene. Her last recorded weight was 72.4 kg about four months prior.

Her current feeding regimen consists of a 2.0 kcal/ml formula at 100 ml/hr for 16 hours (feeding from 1600 to 0800 hours), accompanied by a 120 ml water flush every 4/24 during her 16-hour mealtime, as well as pre and post feeding. This regimen provides 2440 calories, 96 g of protein and 2300 ml of total fluid.

In light of her weight gain, what are some potential considerations and interventions in Amina's case?

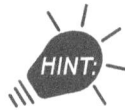

> **HINT:**
>
> Consider recalculating Amina's calorie requirements, evaluating her weight gain in the context of her nutrition status, assessing her activity levels, and consulting with her primary doctor to address fluid retention or medication side effects.

Commentary

Potential considerations

1. **Recalculate calorie requirements:**
    Request an updated weight measurement for Amina, ideally taken in the morning after she has used the bathroom, then re-evaluate her calorie requirements. In the acute phase of a TBI, individuals are known to experience significant hypermetabolism and require 100%–200% of baseline calorie needs.[1] Thus, patients may be discharged from hospital at the upper end of these nutritional requirements, but this needs to be monitored closely once they are back in the community as metabolism plateaus generally happen at two months post injury.[1] There is no specific 'marker' for when metabolism plateaus, but nutritional monitoring may provide some signals that her body is no longer in a state of shock and/or inflammation as it would have been when she was in hospital. Nutritional monitoring may include weight, biochemistry, hand grip strength, and the Subjective Global Assessment (SGA).[2] Refer to Appendix 1 for a visual depiction of the SGA.

2. **Consider Amina's weight gain in the context of her overall nutrition status:**
    Is the 15.4 kg weight gain restoration after previous significant weight loss acquired during her hospital stay?

What is her current body mass index with her weight as it is now, and is this ideal for her? The nutrition intervention best for Amina may include weight maintenance or weight loss depending on whether her current weight is ideal for her or not. It would be relevant to engage her loved ones in this discussion to understand what they think is a healthy weight for Amina, as the body mass index is known to be misleading at times.[3]

3. **Assess Amina's current activity levels:**
    Engage in an in-depth discussion with Amina's family, caregivers and physiotherapist to explore aspects related to mobility and activity levels, and their potential impact on her calorie expenditure. Activity levels, and thus calorie expenditure, may also change with the changing seasons as Amina may be more active in the hotter months and less so in winter. For example, Amina may engage in weekly hydrotherapy in the summer months only, and therefore she may require less feed/fluid during the winter months.

Potential interventions

1. **Reduce calories while maintaining protein and multivitamin intake:**
    One strategy to consider may be to keep Amina on her current formula but reduce the calorie intake by 500 calories or more to create a calorie deficit. Additionally, to ensure she maintains adequate protein intake for muscle mass maintenance, adding protein powder

flushes may be warranted if the drop in calories results in a clinically significant protein intake reduction. It may also be advisable to start Amina on multivitamin or single micronutrient supplementation if the reduction in calories results in her not meeting her recommended daily intake (RDI) of key micronutrients for her age (i.e. iron and calcium).[4]

2. **Switch to a lower calorie, higher protein formula:**
    Transition Amina to a formula with lower calorie content and higher protein content. For instance, consider using a 1.25 kcal/ml formula that provides 64 g of protein per litre. Such a formula would not require the addition of protein powder supplementation and may not require external micronutrient supplementation.

3. **Call for a medical consultation to assess fluid retention and medication side effects:**
    Consult with Amina's primary doctor to investigate the possibility of: 1) fluid retention, 2) medications that may be contributing to the observed weight changes, or 3) thyroid issues contributing to this weight gain. It would also be warranted to request blood tests exploring liver function as well as lipid studies (e.g. triglyceride and cholesterol levels), to ensure any abnormalities that have occurred in conjunction with this significant weight gain are identified and addressed appropriately.[5] Exploring these aspects of Amina's health may be warranted if nutrition interventions to minimise further weight gain are not successful.

4. **Switch to daytime feeding:**

    Research on nightshift workers shows that circadian rhythm disruptions from sleep disturbance and overnight nutrition increase the risk of metabolic diseases and weight gain.[6] This concept applies to adults like Amina who are on continuous overnight tube feeds. Due to the disruption to her circadian rhythm from the continuous overnight feeding, this would disturb her metabolic processes and potentially contribute to her weight gain. Since the body isn't designed to metabolise nutrients efficiently during sleep, gradually transitioning Amina from night-time continuous feeding to daytime continuous or bolus feeding could potentially help reduce weight gain and, coupled with increased activity, could potentially promote weight loss.

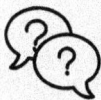

Post-case reflective questions

▶ How would you balance the need to reduce Amina's calorie intake while maintaining her nutritional status?

▶ How would you involve Amina's caregivers in managing her feeding regimen and addressing their concerns about her weight gain?

▶ What medical factors would you explore to rule out other causes of her weight gain (e.g. fluid retention)?

Notes

1. Lee HY and Oh BM (2022, March) 'Nutrition management in patients with traumatic brain injury: A Narrative Review'. *Brain Neurorehabil.* 15(1):e4. doi: 10.12786/bn.2022.15.e4. PMID: 36743843; PMCID: PMC9833460. Available at: https://www.ncbi.nlm.nih.gov/pmc/articles/PMC9833460/

2. Detsky AS, McLaughlin JR, Baker JP, Johnston N, Whittaker S, Mendelson RA & Jeejeebhoy KN (1987) 'What is subjective global assessment of nutritional status?' *JPEN J Parenter Enteral Nutr.* 11(1):8-13. https://doi.org/10.1177/014860718701100108. Available at: https://pubmed.ncbi.nlm.nih.gov/3820522/

3. Rothman KJ (2008) 'BMI-related errors in the measurement of obesity'. *International Journal of Obesity.* 32 Suppl 3:S56-9. doi: 10.1038/ijo.2008.87. PMID: 18695655. Available at: https://pubmed.ncbi.nlm.nih.gov/18695655

4. National Health and Medical Research Council (2021) *Nutrient Reference Values for Australia and New Zealand.* [online] Eatforhealth.gov.au. Available at: https://www.eatforhealth.gov.au/nutrient-reference-values

5. Carmena R, Ascaso JF, Real JT (2001, Oct) 'Impact of obesity in primary hyperlipidemias'. *Nutr Metab Cardiovasc Dis.* 11(5):354-9. PMID: 11887432.

6. Davis C, Huggins CE, Kleve S, Leung GKW, Bonham MP (2024, Feb) 'Conceptualizing weight management for night shift workers: A mixed-methods systematic review'. *Obes Rev.* 25(2):e13659. Available at: https://pubmed.ncbi.nlm.nih.gov/37985937/

Jameel – Assessing Quality of Life

Jameel is a compassionate and determined 39-year-old accountant whose journey is defined by resilience and strength. Despite facing progressive motor neurone disease, which has led to severe dysphagia, Jameel maintains an unwavering spirit and positive outlook on life.

As a result of his dysphagia, Jameel had a feeding tube inserted, a 20 Fr PEG, and was sent home from hospital on four boluses a day on a 1.5 kcal/ml formula. You have been referred to continue Jameel's tube feeding nutrition care in the community. Upon your review, you find he is weight stable and meeting 100% of his calorie and protein needs with no bowel issues.

With no acute nutrition issues identified in your assessment, what approach would you take to evaluate Jameel's quality of life?

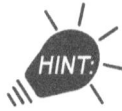

HINT:

Focus on assessing how his feeding regimen impacts his daily activities, mental well-being and social interactions to ensure his quality of life is optimised.

Commentary

Navigating the intricacies of assessing someone's quality of life, particularly when they rely on a home feeding tube, can be profoundly personal and a subjective endeavour.

The very essence of quality of life is deeply individual, making it challenging to capture through standardised measures. An excellent report to read on this topic was prepared by Dr Mercedez Hinchcliff, a researcher at the University of Wollongong (and tubie mum). Her research study exploring the quality of life of home tube-fed Australians showed that 81% of people restrict their social engagements, 50% try to conceal their feeding tubes from their friends, 60% feel excluded from society, and 50% experience depression and anxiety.[1] Sit with those statistics for a bit and let them sink in. As dietitians and clinicians working with this vulnerable population, we can make a difference simply by the energy we bring to a consultation, the information we empower them with to control their own nutrition, and the effective questions we ask.

Home enteral nutrition-specific quality-of-life tools have been developed.[2] While these tools serve as valuable resources for research purposes, their applicability in one-on-one sessions can be limiting. Nonetheless, they can play an important role in sparking ideas and bolstering confidence in clinicians to pose relevant questions about quality of life. So, make sure you read the references listed for this case![1,2,3,4]

Some suggested questions to ask Jameel to explore his quality of life with his current feeding regimen include:

► "Do you find yourself changing your social plans based on your feeding schedule?"

► "Has tube feeding impacted your social engagements?"

► "When you are preparing for a day out, how do you pack your tube feeding equipment? Let's see if we can help make any aspect of it easier."

► "When your partner gives you your bolus feed, do you find it bothersome to have someone standing over you during the feed? Perhaps setting a pump for the bolus feed may give you more autonomy and allow you to sit at the meal table with your family."

Starting with direct queries, requiring simple yes or no responses or referencing specific aspects of the tube feeding experience, can serve as a practical approach. Alternatively, more open-ended questions like "What did you do over the weekend?" can potentially unveil subtle cues indicating potential social withdrawal due to tube feeding or bowel issues.

The bottom line is to be careful to not assume that achieving 100% of calorie, protein and fluid needs, coupled with bowel control and weight stability, necessarily translate into a high quality of life and happiness for Jameel. As a clinician, you must skilfully navigate the landscape of asking nuanced questions to effectively evaluate quality of life amidst the clinical needs of your clients. Don't overthink it; be human and authentic in your approach.

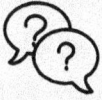

> ## Post-case reflective questions
>
> ► How would you evaluate the impact of Jameel's feeding regimen on his social life and emotional well-being?
>
> ► What would you prioritise if Jameel expressed a desire for more autonomy in managing his feeding schedule?

Notes

1. Hinchcliff M Dr (2023) *Summary of Survey Results | Health-related quality of life in patients who utilise home enteral nutrition in Australia/New Zealand*. ausEE Inc. and the University of Wollongong. [online] Available at: https://feedingtubeaware.com.au/abouttubefeeding/research/

2. Cuerda MC, Apezetxea A, Carrillo L, Casanueva F, Cuesta F, Irles JA, Virgili MN, Layola M and Lizan L (2016 Nov 4) 'Development and validation of a specific questionnaire to assess health-related quality of life in patients with home enteral nutrition: NutriQoL® development'. *Patient Prefer Adherence*. 10:2289-2296. doi: 10.2147/PPA.S110188. PMID: 27853360; PMCID: PMC5104289. Available at: https://www.ncbi.nlm.nih.gov/pmc/articles/PMC5104289/

3. Stevens CS, Lemon B, Lockwood GA, Waldron JN, Bezjak A and Ringash J (2011 Aug) 'The development and validation of a quality-of-life questionnaire for head and neck cancer patients with enteral feeding tubes: the QOL-EF'. *Supportive Care in Cancer*. 19(8):1175-82. doi: 10.1007/s00520-010-0934-6. Epub 2010 Jun 24. PMID: 20574664. Available at: https://pubmed.ncbi.nlm.nih.gov/20574664/

4. Chen C, Zhu D, Zhao Z and Ye X (2022 Aug) 'Quality of life assessment instruments in adult patients receiving home parenteral and enteral nutrition: A scoping review'. *Nutr Clin Pract*. 37(4):811-824. doi: 10.1002/ncp.10848. Epub 2022 Mar 2. PMID: 35235230. Available at: https://pubmed.ncbi.nlm.nih.gov/35235230/

Harpreet – Homemade Blends

Harpreet is a 67-year-old man who was discharged from hospital with a PEG tube after losing the ability to swallow on the background of Parkinson's disease. He cherishes moments spent enjoying his favourite pastimes, such as fishing and cricket, finding solace and camaraderie in these activities.

Harpreet has a 24 Fr (4.5cm shaft length), low-profile gastrostomy tube anchored in place with a balloon (fill volume of 7 ml water). His feeding regimen is four bolus tube feeds per day at 0930, 1230, 1600 and 1930 of 2.0 kcal/ml formula with 100 ml of water pre and post each bolus. He connects a

60 cm extension set to his low-profile tube and then attaches that to a 60 ml syringe for gravity bolus feeds.

His wife enquires about putting traditional curry meals through his PEG.

How would you manage this request? Jot down the thoughts running through your mind.

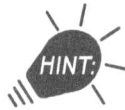

HINT:

Embrace the opportunity to explore effective and safe ways to accommodate Harpreet's wife's enquiry and curiosity to help her husband enjoy traditional meals while prioritising his feeding tube's wellbeing.

Commentary

Managing Harpreet's wife's request to put traditional curry meals through his PEG tube involves considering several important factors to ensure administration efficiency, nutritional needs are met, and the functionality of the PEG tube. Here are some considerations:

1. **Consistency of the blends:**

   ▸ Traditional curry consistency may not be the right viscosity for administration into a 24 Fr PEG tube. It would need to be pureed to a smooth consistency with no lumps and potentially strained. An important consideration would be to teach Harpreet's wife to test the viscosity of the blend for feeding tube appropriateness using an objective measure, such as the International Dysphagia Diet Standardisation Initiative (IDDSI) Syringe Flow Test.[2]

2. **Nutritional adequacy:**

   ▸ It's important to determine if the homemade blends will be Harpreet's sole source of nutrition or just an occasional family meal. This will guide the extent to which the blends need to be nutritionally balanced and consistent with his current feeding regimen.

   ▸ The current formula Harpreet is on is a 2.0 kcal/ml high-calorie formula. Replicating this calorie concentration with homemade food can be challenging but not impossible.

3. **Tube patency:**

   ▶ Proper cleaning of the feeding tube is essential, and his current regimen includes 100 ml of water pre and post each bolus feed. This practice would need to be maintained and possibly increased to more water flushing more frequently to ensure no food residue remains in the tube.

4. **Hygiene and food safety:**

   ▶ Home-prepared tube feeding blends must be handled and stored safely to avoid contamination and infection, just like one would with regular meal preparation. This includes preparing food in a clean environment, storing it at the correct temperature, cooking food thoroughly, using separate chopping boards for meats and vegetable, and following proper hand hygiene practices during preparation.[1]

5. **Consulting other healthcare professionals:**

   ▶ Informing Harpreet's healthcare team, including his gastroenterologist and general practitioner, is important to ensure that all team members are on the same page regarding his nutrition.

▶ If Harpreet has a community nurse supporting his tube feeding care and stoma site care, they should also be informed of this transition.

6. Educational support:

▶ Preparing home-cooked tube feeding blends in a manner suitable for PEG tube feeding can be time-consuming and labour-intensive. Assess whether Harpreet's wife is comfortable with this and able to commit to this additional task.

▶ Provide comprehensive training to Harpreet's wife on how to prepare the meals, blend them, strain them and administer them through the PEG tube safely.

▶ Instead of blending existing curry recipes, Harpreet's wife may prefer to work with you to create tube feeding-friendly recipes that include several cultural ingredients.

7. Equipment support:

▶ Some tube feeding equipment that is unique to using homemade blends as formula are:

  ▪ Blender: An appropriate blender is essential for achieving a smooth, lump-free consistency suitable for tube feeding. The blender should be powerful enough to thoroughly blend all ingredients to a fine texture.

  ▪ O-Ring syringes: These syringes are recommended for their durability and ease of use. They provide a reliable and efficient way to administer the blended formula through the PEG tube.[3] O-ring syringes also tend to have a smoother plunger action, making feeding more comfortable and manageable.

- Straight connector extension sets: Straight connector extension sets are preferred over right-angled ones as they allow for a more direct and unobstructed flow of the blended formula.[3]

8. Monitoring and evaluation:

▶ Establish a monitoring plan to check Harpreet's weight, hydration status and overall health to ensure the new feeding regimen is nutritionally sound. You may consider checking his nutrition bloods (e.g. iron studies, B12, folate, vitamin D) pre-commencement and then 6–12 months into the new regimen.[3]

When supporting Harpreet with homemade blends, it's important to remember that the effects of blended tube feeding versus conventional commercial formulas, particularly in relation to adverse events like tube blockages in adults, remains limited.[4] While more research is needed to fully understand the impact of homemade blended tube feeding on clinical outcomes, there are numerous resources available from reputable organisations like ASPEN (American Society for Parenteral and Enteral Nutrition), BDA (British Dietetic Association), and AuSPEN (Australasian Society of Parenteral and Enteral Nutrition) to help guide you in safely empowering Harpreet to transition to homemade blended tube feeding. [1,3,5]

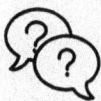

Post-case reflective questions

▶ How would you ensure that the homemade blends meet Harpreet's nutritional needs and maintain his tube's functionality?

▶ What steps would you take to train Harpreet's wife in preparing and administering homemade blends safely?

Notes

1. Australasian Society of Parenteral and Enteral Nutrition (AuSPEN) (2021, July) *Blended tube feeding in enteral feeding: Consensus Statement.* [online] https://custom.cvent.com/FE8ADE3646EB4896BCEA8239F12DC577/ files/3ba20002ad1e4837881ab92135d57458.pdf. Available at: https:// www.auspen.org.au/resources-1

2. *Drink Testing Methods* (n.d.) International Dysphagia Diet Standardisation Initiative (IDDSI). https://iddsi.org/framework/drink-testing-methods

3. Epp L, Blackmer AB, Church A, Ford I, Grenda B, Larimer C, Lewis-Ayalloore J, Malone A, Pataki L, Rempel G and Washington V (2023) 'Blenderized tube feedings: Practice recommendations from the American Society for Parenteral and Enteral Nutrition'. *Nutrition in Clinical Practice*, 38(6), pp.1190–1219. doi:https://doi.org/10.1002/ ncp.11055. Available at: https://aspenjournals.onlinelibrary.wiley.com/ doi/abs/10.1002/ncp.11055

4. Breik L, Barker L, Bauer J and Davidson Z (2023, December) 'Blended tube feeding formula compared to conventional formula in adults on enteral nutrition: A systematic review'. *Nutrition and Dietetics*. 2024;1-16. doi:10.1111/1747-0080.1291216. Available at: https://onlinelibrary.wiley. com/doi/10.1111/1747-0080.12912

5. British Dietetic Association (n.d.) *Launch of BDA Practice Toolkit: The Use of Blended Diet with Enteral Feeding Tubes.* [online] www.bda.uk.com. Available at: https://www.bda.uk.com/resource/launch-of-bda-practice-toolkit-the-use-of-blended-diet-with-enteral-feeding-tubes.html

Sakina –
Fostering
Independence

Sakina, an 18-year-old woman with cerebral palsy (Spastic Quadriplegia), has a big hearty laugh that those around her adore. She relies on a low-profile gastrostomy tube for her nutritional needs.

Her nutritional intake consists of a 1.0 kcal/ml formula with a total daily formula volume of 1500 ml, divided into four mealtimes per day. At each mealtime, her mother connects a 30 cm extension set to her button and administers 375ml of the formula with 50 ml of water before and after each meal through a 60 ml syringe via gravity. Each meal takes around 15–20 minutes.

With an aim to foster more independence for Sakina now that she is an adult, how can you and her caregivers work collaboratively to empower Sakina in managing aspects of her nutrition and daily life, considering her unique challenges?

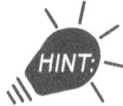

> **HINT:**
>
> Consider strategies that allow Sakina to participate more in her feeding process as well as enable opportunities to network with other tubies.

Lina Breik

Commentary

To enhance Sakina's autonomy in managing her nutrition and daily life, several strategies can be implemented with consideration given to her abilities, cerebral palsy and reliance on a feeding tube.

By focusing on these strategies, Sakina can gain more independence and confidence in managing her nutritional needs and daily activities.

1. Optimise tube feeding equipment:

    ▸ Explore using a 60 cm extension set for Sakina's gastrostomy tube instead of the standard 30 cm to avoid Sakina having someone standing over her at mealtimes. Also, with Spastic Quadriplegia, spastic movements in the arms are common, which may be difficult to manage with a shorter extension set.

    ▸ Introduce tube feeding mobility-enhancing equipment to improve portability of her tube feeding supplies. Examples of innovative ways to support this include the Mobility+[1] or FreeArm[2] backpacks available through Tube Fun.[3]

    ▸ Opt for more portable formula packaging by switching to 125 ml or 200 ml bottles instead of the larger 500 ml or 1000 ml bottles.

    ▸ Personalise the look of Sakina's feeding tube and stoma site with colourful patches, belts and bags, contributing to a positive and empowering experience. Check out Tubie Fun for more ideas of bringing fun and laughter to tubie equipment.[3]

2. **Empowerment through choice:**
   Evaluate the feasibility of incorporating both continuous and bolus pump feeds into Sakina's regimen, enabling her to adapt her mealtimes to her daily activities and promoting greater autonomy. Empower her by allowing choices about her feeding regimen, such as selecting the times for her mealtimes and deciding on comfortable positions during her mealtimes.

3. **Encourage community connection:**
   Connect Sakina with online support groups tailored to individuals with feeding tubes. AusEE Inc. is an Australian not-for-profit organisation that leads Feeding Tube Awareness Week annually and regularly hosts virtual support groups for people with feeding tubes.[4,5] Other avenues available to explore the tubie community include reading The Blend magazine.[6]

4. **Learn communication techniques:**
   Collaborate with a speech pathologist and her caregivers to implement a communication board tailored to Sakina's needs if she doesn't already have one. This would enhance her ability to express preferences and actively participate in decision-making regarding her nutrition as much as possible.

5. **Mealtime companionship:**

   Check in with Sakina and her mother about their mealtime companionship preferences at social events. Determine if Sakina enjoys sharing mealtime with family and friends at the dinner table or if she prefers setting up a feeding pump discreetly in the background.

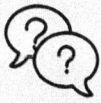

Post-case reflective questions

► How would you balance Sakina's desire for autonomy with ensuring her safety during mealtimes?

► What role could her caregivers play in supporting her journey towards greater independence?

Notes

1. Rockfieldmd.com (n.d.) *Rockfield MD*. [online] Available at: https://rockfieldmd.com/ [Accessed 18 Sep. 2024]

2. FreeArm (n.d.) *FreeArm*. [online] Available at: https://freearmcare.com/ [Accessed 18 Sep. 2024]

3. Tubie Fun (n.d.) *Tubie Fun*. [online] Available at: https://tubiefun.com.au/ [Accessed 18 Sep. 2024]

4. ausEE Inc. (n.d.) *ausEE Inc*. [online] Available at: https://www.ausee.org/ [Accessed 18 Sep. 2024]

5. Feeding Tube Aware. (2024) *Feeding Tube Awareness Week*. [online] Available at: https://www.feedingtubeaware.com.au/ [Accessed 18 Sep. 2024]

6. The Blend (2024) *The Blend*. [online] Available at: https://www.theblendmag.com/ [Accessed 18 Sep. 2024]

Case 13

Aziba – Wound Healing

Aziba, a 48-year-old mother of a policeman, has progressive multiple sclerosis. The progressive nature of her condition has significantly impacted her swallowing ability, leaving her dependent on a RIG feeding tube for nutritional support. Despite these challenges, Aziba remains positive and always has a warm smile and a joke ready to lift everyone's spirits.

Aziba recently developed a pressure injury (stage II) on her sacrum. The only nutrition-related information you have about her includes:

► Weight – 62kg, body mass index – 26kg/m².

► Orally managing a pureed diet and thickened fluids (supporting 50% of her nutritional needs).

- ► Through her RIG she administers a 1.5 kcal/ml fibre-containing formula as 250ml boluses twice a day (100 ml water before and after each). This provides ~32 g protein and 750 calories.

How might you enhance the healing of her wound through nutritional intervention?

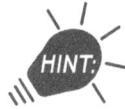

> *HINT:*
>
> Consider supporting Aziba's wound healing with a protein-rich tube feeding regimen and/or wound healing supplements, and close collaboration with other professionals for optimal pressure relief.

Commentary

Here are some strategies to enhance wound healing from a nutrition perspective:

1. **Increase protein intake:**
    Aziba is currently receiving 1.0 g/kg of protein, assuming 50% of her needs are being met orally and 50% through her RIG. To support wound healing an intake of 1.25–1.5 g/kg/day for adults is recommended.[1] Given that Aziba is slightly above her healthy body mass index range, you want to increase her protein intake without increasing calorie intake too much. This can be achieved by:

    a. Fortifying her oral diet to include protein-rich foods at mealtimes or high-protein thickened oral supplements between mealtimes.

    b. Selecting a formula with an elevated protein content and lower calorie content such as a 1.25 kcal/ml formulation with ~60–65 g protein in 1000 ml of formula.

    c. Incorporating protein powder supplements into the RIG feeding routine. Practically, this could be two scoops of a protein powder three times a day mixed in 120 ml (or more/less depending on the manufacturer's instruction and hydration needs) of water each time and syringed into her feeding tube between main mealtimes. Six scoops a day of such a protein powder could provide an additional ~20 g of protein (extra protein amount depends on the brand of the protein powder selected).

2. **Introduce a specific wound healing supplement:**
    Consider supplementing Aziba's tube feeding regimen with a specific wound healing powder that contains arginine, zinc and antioxidants. Such powders often come in sachets or in a tin. They can be added to Aziba's oral foods or into her RIG regimen dissolved in a water flush as per the manufacturer's recommendations. Evidence corroborates their effectiveness in increasing the rate of wound healing in those with baseline adequate protein intake and those who are malnourished and/or at risk of malnutrition. They ideally should be taken for a period of at least four weeks for maximum benefit. [1]

3. **Monitor bowel output:**
    Pay careful attention to Aziba's bowel output, assessing colour, frequency and consistency. Any excessively loose stools can spill into the wound resulting in a potential infection and delayed healing. Loose stools can be managed through adequate fibre intake, hydration and/or medication strategies. A temporary faecal containment device may be warranted in situations where a person has chronic loose stools hindering wound healing of a sacral pressure injury.[2]

4. **Optimise pressure relief:**

   Ensure Aziba is well supported by other healthcare professionals who can contribute to assessing optimal pressure relief equipment for the affected area. An occupational therapist, for example, can recommend specialised cushions or mattresses.

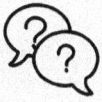

Post-case reflective questions

► What key factors would you monitor to ensure Aziba's wound heals properly while meeting her nutritional needs?

► How would you adapt her feeding plan to address the specific challenges of wound healing?

► What other healthcare professionals would you collaborate with to support her recovery?

Notes

1. Munoz N, Posthauer ME, Cereda E, Schols JMGA and Haesler E
   (2020) 'The Role of Nutrition for Pressure Injury Prevention and
   Healing'. *Advances in Skin & Wound Care*, [online] 33(3), pp.123–136.
   doi:https://doi.org/10.1097/01.asw.0000653144.90739.ad. Available at:
   https://journals.lww.com/aswcjournal/fulltext/2020/03000/the_role_of_
   nutrition_for_pressure_injury.3.aspx

2. Ousey K and Gillibrand W (2010) 'Using faecal collectors to reduce
   wound contamination'. *Wounds*. 6(1). https://wounds-uk.com/wp-
   content/uploads/sites/2/2023/02/content_9343.pdf

Patricia – Continuous to Bolus with Insulin

Patricia, a lively 62-year-old retired pharmacist, recently faced a significant health challenge with a sudden left frontal stroke.

Despite this, her spirit remains strong as she navigates life with a RIG feeding tube. This tube, a size 22 Fr with a 3.5 cm skin-level marking on the external skin disc, supports her with a continuous 16-hour infusion of a 1.5 kcal/ml formula at 75 ml/hr from 0800 to 0000.

Living with insulin-dependent type 2 diabetes mellitus, Patricia maintains good control of her blood sugar, with her last haemoglobin A1C (HbA1c) at 6.3%. Ever proactive about her health and quality of life, Patricia is keen to switch to a bolus daytime feeding regimen, which would grant her more mobility and freedom during the day.

How would you go about helping her make the transition?

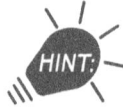

> **HINT:**
>
> Explore strategies to support Patricia's transition to a bolus daytime feeding regimen, emphasising collaboration with her endocrinologist and careful planning to ensure the safe and smooth transition of her feeding regimen, avoiding any hypoglycaemic episodes.

Lina Breik

Commentary

Transitioning Patricia from a continuous feeding regimen to a bolus daytime feeding regimen requires careful planning and monitoring.

Here are key considerations to ensure a safe transition:

1. **Understand Patricia's preferences for the number of mealtimes according to her daily routine:**
   Determine the number of boluses Patricia prefers and the timing for each mealtime to align with her daily routine.

2. **Divide her formula volume needs by the number of mealtimes per day:**
   Calculate the total daily volume of the formula and divide it into several bolus mealtimes. Her current 1200 ml of formula per day can be split into five mealtimes of 240 ml formula each feed. You may consider switching her to a more concentrated 2.0 kcal/ml formula, which would mean she can have four mealtimes instead at 240 ml each feed (960 ml formula volume). The volume of formula given per mealtime can be more than 240 ml depending on her tolerance to higher volumes. Remember, 240 ml is just under one cup!

3. **Review her insulin regimen and coordinate with her endocrinologist:**
   Understand Patricia's current insulin regimen, including whether she uses slow- or fast-acting insulin and the timing and dosage of all medications. You should also work with her endocrinologist to adjust her insulin regimen, modifying both the dose and timing according to her new feeding regimen to prevent hypo- or hyperglycaemia. Send a detailed letter outlining the proposed changes to her regimen to her endocrinologist, including a breakdown of her carbohydrate distribution compared to the previous plan.

4. **Remember to ensure fibre in her formula:**
   Ensure she is on a fibre-containing formula to help maintain blood glucose levels effectively.[1]

5. **Hypoglycaemia management preparedness is very important for safety:**
   Ensure Patricia and her primary caregiver are educated on hypoglycaemia management, recognising signs and knowing how to provide immediate treatment.

6. **Create a transition plan:**
   Start on a Monday when her endocrinologist is available to troubleshoot any immediate insulin dosage adjustments required. Here's a sample plan:

   ▶ Days 1–4: Switch to a 2.0 kcal/ml formula and run for eight hours at 120 ml/hr (totalling 960 ml). This reduces feeding time and tests her tolerance to a higher volume of formula administration. Adjust insulin to the new carbohydrate distribution with her endocrinologist.

► Days 5–7: Introduce a 120 ml bolus at 0800 via gravity syringe, followed by continuous pump feeding from 1000 to 1700 at 120 ml/hr. Administer rapid-acting insulin immediately after the bolus, matching the nutrition and insulin.[2]

► Days 8–ongoing: Introduce a 190 ml bolus at 0800. If tolerated, continue with 190 ml boluses at 1000, 1300, 1500 and 1800, totalling 950 ml daily. Administer rapid-acting insulin after each bolus, noting that a 190 ml bolus of a 2.0 kcal/ml formula provides ~42–55g of carbohydrate per mealtime.

► If Patricia wants to reduce mealtimes further to four boluses a day, increase the volume administered to 240ml at 0800, 1300, 1500 and 1800 supported by rapid-acting insulin after each mealtime.

7. **Develop a contingency plan if Patricia vomits:**
   In the event that Patricia vomits during the transition regimen, collaborate with her endocrinologist to decide on the best course of action in the context of her prescribed insulin. She may need to be started on slow pump-administered feeds at, for example, her usual tolerated rate of 75 ml/hr for a few hours straight after her vomit to prevent a hypoglycaemic episode.

8. **Continuous monitoring:**
Encourage Patricia to monitor her blood glucose levels closely throughout the transition (e.g. upon waking up, midday, late afternoon and before bed), record them, and book in a review consultation with her endocrinologist to adjust insulin dosage as necessary.

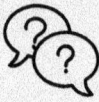

Post-case reflective questions

▶ How would you ensure Patricia's blood glucose levels remain stable while transitioning to bolus feeding?

▶ What challenges might arise during this transition, and how would you prepare for them?

▶ How would you involve her endocrinologist in the process to ensure a smooth adjustment in her insulin regimen?

Notes

1. Xie Y, Gou L, Peng M, Zheng J and Chen L (2020) 'Effects of soluble fiber supplementation on glycemic control in adults with type 2 diabetes mellitus: A systematic review and meta-analysis of randomized controlled trials'. *Clinical Nutrition.* https://doi.org/10.1016/j.clnu.2020.10.032. Available at: https://www.clinicalnutritionjournal.com/article/S0261-5614(20)30575-6/abstract

2. Mabrey ME, Barton AB, Corsino L, Freeman SB, Davis ED, Bell EL and Setji TL (2015) 'Managing hyperglycemia and diabetes in patients receiving enteral feedings: A health system approach'. *Hospital Practice*, 43(2), 74–78. https://doi.org/10.1080/21548331.2015.1022493. Available at: https://www.ncbi.nlm.nih.gov/pmc/articles/PMC4397647

Case 15

Rana – Bolus to Continuous

Rana is a 56-year-old retired teacher with Parkinson's disease. Diagnosed several years ago, she has been managing her condition effectively with medication up until three months ago. A new challenge presented itself when she lost the ability to swallow food safely, and she now has a feeding tube.

Rana relies on four PEG boluses (~0900, 1130, 1530, 1800) of a 1.5 kcal/ml formula. This routine, while providing essential nourishment, has begun to encroach on her daily activities and mental space. In a recent conversation with you, Rana expressed a desire for a more convenient feeding schedule that would allow her to minimise constant interactions and thoughts about her PEG.

What factors may be considered when addressing her request?

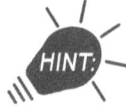

HINT:

Think about adjusting the frequency, volume and timing of Rana's mealtimes to minimise constant interactions with her PEG tube during the day and improve her mental well-being while meeting her nutritional needs.

Commentary

Your considerations may include:

1. **Duration and timing of current feeding:**
   Explore the reasons why the boluses impact her ability to engage in other activities throughout the day. Is it the time of the boluses? Duration of a mealtime? Fear of feeding in public? Current tube feeding equipment not portable enough to support an active life?

2. **Feed delivery method:**
   Is Rana currently having her mealtime boluses via pump, gravity-set drip or syringe? Rana could be trained in all three delivery methods to allow her the flexibility to choose what suits her best for a particular day based on her activities.

3. **Daily schedule and activities:**
   Evaluate Rana's daily schedule and activities to develop a feeding regimen that aligns with her lifestyle. For example, on the days she has several activities during the day time which may hinder her ability to have the first three boluses of the day, she may choose to have one mealtime upon waking up, and then make up the remaining volume of formula in the evenings via pump over a 2–4-hour period. For example, she could run the pump at 250 ml per hour for three hours for a total of 750 ml of a 2.0 kcal/

ml formula, which would provide 62 g protein and 1500 calories.

4. **Formula:**

   Explore the option of transitioning Rana to a more concentrated formula, such as a 2.0 kcal/ml. While still meeting her nutritional needs, this adjustment could potentially allow for a reduction in the volume and increase in the speed of each PEG feed bolus. Another option would be to consider a 1.5 kcal/ml or 2.0 kcal/ml formula that is packaged in a portable 125 ml or 200 ml bottle for ease of mobility out of the home.

5. **Drug-nutrient interactions:**

   Consider the timing of Rana's Parkinson's medication. Ensure that the new feeding schedule is away from medication times to minimise any potential drug-nutrient interactions. A high-protein diet may reduce the therapeutic effect of some Parkinson's medications.[1]

6. **Hydration management:**

   Consider Rana's hydration needs and encourage her to distribute fluid intake throughout the day to prevent an excessive amount of fluid intake in the evening which could impact her sleep quality.

7. **Psychosocial impact:**

   Consider the psychosocial impact of the feeding regimen on Rana's mental and emotional well-being. Research shows that 81% of adults with a feeding tube limit their social engagements, 50% hide their feeding tube from friends, 60% feel excluded from social activities, and 50% experience depression and anxiety.[2] It's important to address these aspects of Rana's request and refer her for psychological support if needed.

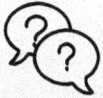

Post-case reflective questions

► How would you assess whether continuous feeding is the best option for Rana's comfort and nutritional needs?

► How would you monitor the success of this transition in terms of both nutritional intake and quality of life?

► What are the potential benefits and risks of continuous feeding compared to bolus feeding?

Notes

1. Agnieszka W, Paweł P and Małgorzata K (2022, April 21) 'How to Optimize the Effectiveness and Safety of Parkinson's Disease Therapy? - A Systematic Review of Drugs Interactions with Food and Dietary Supplements'. *Curr Neuropharmacol.* 20(7):1427-1447. doi: 10.2174/15 70159X19666211116142806. PMID: 34784871; PMCID: PMC9881082. Available at: https://pubmed.ncbi.nlm.nih.gov/34784871/

2. Hinchcliff M Dr (2023) Summary of Survey Results | *Health-related quality of life in patients who utilise home enteral nutrition in Australia/New Zealand.* ausEE Inc. and the University of Wollongong. [online] Available at: https://feedingtubeaware.com.au/abouttubefeeding/research/

Case 16

Belinda – Advanced Dementia

Belinda is a 75-year-old woman bravely navigating the advanced stages of dementia. Recently, she's lost all interest in eating, which is a common, though challenging, part of this journey. Despite the doctors' guidance suggesting a limited life expectancy and recognising the natural progression of her condition, Belinda's husband can't bear the thought of her suffering from hunger. Belinda does not have medical decision-making capacity, and out of his deep concern for her, her husband decided that Belinda should have a feeding tube inserted to ensure she receives nutrition.

During your follow-up visit to Belinda's home to review her tube feeding nutrition care, you discover that her husband, with the best of intentions, has been overfeeding her by 50% of her calorie needs.

How do you handle this situation? Write down a few words or sentences you'd incorporate in your discussion with her husband.

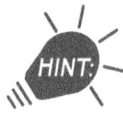

> **HINT:**
>
> Consider addressing the husband's concerns with empathy, while educating him about the risks of overfeeding.

Commentary

Approaching this delicate situation requires a blend of empathy, clear communication and education. Here's a thoughtful approach for consideration:

1. **Establish a compassionate connection:**
    Begin by expressing understanding and empathy for the husband's concerns. Acknowledge his love and dedication to Belinda's well-being, for example, "I can see how much you care about Belinda, and your commitment to her health is truly admirable."

2. **Educate about nutritional needs:**
    Gently explain the importance of proper nutritional care for individuals with advanced dementia, and let him know that you both share a common goal for Belinda to be well nourished and hydrated. However, highlight how overfeeding can be harmful and lead to complications such as aspiration pneumonia, gastrointestinal discomfort and metabolic imbalances. You might say, "While it's natural to want to give Belinda as much nutrition as possible, her body can only handle a certain amount. Too many calories can actually cause her discomfort and health issues."

3. **Discuss the feeding tube's purpose:**
    Clarify the role of the feeding tube in providing comfort rather than prolonging life in a burdensome way. Reinforce that the goal is to ensure Belinda's comfort and

quality of life, for example, "The feeding tube is here to make sure Belinda is comfortable and not suffering from hunger, but it's not meant to force her body to take in more than it needs or more than it can handle."

4. **Offer practical guidance:**

Provide a clear, revised feeding plan that aligns with Belinda's calorie needs. This plan should be simple and easy for her husband to follow, for example, something as simple as "Based on Belinda's current needs, we should aim for 1300 ml of the 1.25 kcal/ml formula daily. I'll provide a detailed feeding regimen to help guide you on how to give her this nutrition."

5. **Reassure ongoing support:**

Reassure the husband that you and the healthcare team are there to support him and Belinda throughout this process. Encourage them to reach out with any questions or concerns. You could say, "We're here to support you every step of the way. Please don't hesitate to reach out if you notice any changes or have any concerns about Belinda's care."

6. **Address emotional concerns:**

Be prepared to listen to the husband's emotional concerns and offer advice or resources, such as counselling or support groups, to help him cope with this challenging time. Collaborating with Belinda's primary medical doctor would also be pivotal in ensuring a cohesive and comprehensive care plan and providing a united front in supporting Belinda's well-being.

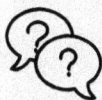

Post-case reflective questions

▶ How would you involve Belinda's caregivers in making decisions about her feeding regimen as her condition progresses?

▶ How would you assess her quality of life and make recommendations to ensure she remains comfortable?

Recommended reading

1. Ijaopo EO and Ijaopo RO (2019) 'Tube Feeding in Individuals with Advanced Dementia: A Review of Its Burdens and Perceived Benefits'. *Journal of Aging Research*. 2019:7272067. doi: 10.1155/2019/7272067. PMID: 31929906; PMCID: PMC6942829. Available at: https://www.ncbi.nlm.nih.gov/pmc/articles/PMC6942829/

2. Schwartz DB, Barrocas A, Annetta MG, Stratton K, McGinnis C, Hardy G, Wong T, Arenas D, Turon-Findley MP, Kliger RG, Corkins KG, Mirtallo J, Amagai T and Guenter, P (2021) 'Ethical Aspects of Artificially Administered Nutrition and Hydration: An ASPEN Position Paper'. *Nutrition in Clinical Practice*, 36(2), pp.254–267. doi:https://doi.org/10.1002/ncp.10633. Available at: https://aspenjournals.onlinelibrary.wiley.com/doi/10.1002/ncp.10633

Case 17

Zichen – Post-Prandial Hypotension

Zichen, a resilient 64-year-old gentleman who was recently diagnosed with progressive supranuclear palsy, now relies on a RIG tube for his nourishment (16 Fr in size).

Zichen's daily routine includes three 200 ml boluses of a 2.0 kcal/ml fibre-rich formula. Each mealtime is supplemented with 50 ml of water before and after, bringing his total fluid intake to 900 ml over 24 hours. He's managing to maintain a stable weight and is comfortably within his healthy weight range.

Recently, Zichen's son has noticed that after each bolus feed, his blood pressure takes a nosedive, causing him to feel lightheaded, sleepy and nauseous.

What additional questions would you consider asking Zichen and his son to get to the root of the problem?

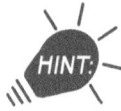

HINT:

Consider asking whether Zichen is on fluid restriction or not. Explore dehydration signs and review recent medical assessments, medication reviews, and blood glucose level checks.

Lina Breik

Commentary

Zichen is likely experiencing post-prandial hypotension (PPH), a condition where blood pressure drops significantly after eating. This condition is prevalent in up to 75% of older people on tube feeding. [1,2]

Additional questions to ask

1. **Hydration and electrolytes:**

   ► Is Zichen on a fluid restriction for any reason?

   ► Does Zichen have any signs of dehydration, such as dark yellow, foul-smelling urine?

   ► Is there a possibility of dehydration or electrolyte imbalance?

2. **Timing and pattern of symptoms:**

   ► When did these symptoms start?

   ► Do the symptoms occur immediately after the bolus feed or at a certain time afterward?

   ► Are the symptoms consistent with each feed or the same time each day, or do they vary?

3. **Details of feeding process:**

   ► How quickly is each bolus administered?

   ► Has there been any recent change in the formula or the amount of water used?

4. **Physical activity and blood glucose levels:**

  ▶ Is there any physical activity or movement that follows the feeding which could influence his symptoms?

  ▶ Have Zichen's blood glucose levels been checked during these episodes of drowsiness and nausea?

5. **Medications and other health issues:**

  ▶ Has there been any change in his medication regimen recently?

    ▪ Has he had recent changes in his blood pressure medications or diuretics?

  ▶ Is he experiencing any other symptoms or health issues that coincide with these episodes?

Potential solutions

1. **Formula adjustment:**

  ▶ Switch to a lower concentration formula, such as a 1.25 kcal/ml or a 1.5 kcal/ml, to increase fluid intake.

2. **Increase fluid intake:**

  ▶ Introduce additional water flushes throughout the day and increase the pre/post bolus water flush amount to provide a total of at least 2.0 L/day.[3]

3. **Feeding schedule adjustment:**

    1. One reported strategy to improve PPH is having six small meals compared to three large meals.[4] So, instead of three boluses during the day through his feeding tube, aim for six to nine smaller boluses.

    2. Another option could be to consider switching to pump feeding to provide a more gradual, consistent flow of nutrition and hydration which may help keep his blood pressure stable.[2]

4. **Sodium content:**

    ▸ Explore the sodium content of the formula and liaise with his primary doctor to determine if an increase in sodium intake would be beneficial.

It's important to run any potential interventions you want to try with Zichen by his primary doctor, and make sure there is medical follow-up of his blood pressure readings a few days after whatever solution you intend to implement.

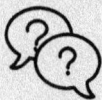

Post-case reflective questions

► What strategies could you implement to reduce the likelihood of Zichen experiencing post-prandial hypotension after his mealtimes?

► How would you collaborate with Zichen's doctor to ensure his PPH is being managed effectively?

Notes

1. Sato K, Sugiura T, Ohte N and Dohi Y (2018) 'Postprandial hypotension in older people receiving tube feeding through gastrostomy'. *Geriatrics & Gerontology International*, 18(10), pp.1474–1478. doi:https://doi.org/10.1111/ggi.13515. Available at: https://onlinelibrary.wiley.com/doi/10.1111/ggi.13515

2. Lubart E, Segal R, Baumoehl Y, Matron M and Leibovitz A (2006) 'Postprandial Hypotension in Long-Term Care Elderly Patients on Enteral Feeding'. *Journal of the American Geriatrics Society*, 54(9), pp.1377–1381. doi:https://doi.org/10.1111/j.1532-5415.2006.00839.x. Available at: https://agsjournals.onlinelibrary.wiley.com/doi/10.1111/j.1532-5415.2006.00839.x

3. Volkert D, Beck AM, Cederholm T, Cruz-Jentoft A, Goisser S, Hooper L, Kiesswetter E, Maggio M, Raynaud-Simon A, Sieber CC, Sobotka L, van Asselt D, Wirth R and Bischoff SC (2019) 'ESPEN guideline on clinical nutrition and hydration in geriatrics'. *Clinical Nutrition*. 38(1):10-47. doi: 10.1016/j.clnu.2018.05.024. PMID: 30005900. Available at: https://pubmed.ncbi.nlm.nih.gov/30005900/

4. Awosika A, Adabanya U, Millis RM, Omole AE and Moon JH (2023, Feb 24) 'Postprandial Hypotension: An Underreported Silent Killer in the Aged'. *Cureus*. 15(2):e35411. doi: 10.7759/cureus.35411. PMID: 36851946; PMCID: PMC9964048. doi:https://doi.org/10.7759/cureus.35411. Available at: https://www.cureus.com/articles/140313-postprandial-hypotension-an-underreported-silent-killer-in-the-aged#!/

Jovana – Regurgitation

Jovana, a vibrant 35-year-old with a passion for cats, is losing her ability to swallow on the background of spinal muscular atrophy (type 4). Jovana uses a PEG tube (16 Fr) to meet half of her nutrition and hydration needs. Her feeding tube is anchored with a 6 ml water-filled balloon.

Jovana currently receives 200 ml three times a day of a 1.5 kcal/ml formula, in addition to oral intake between boluses. She is allowed a minced and moist diet orally.

At your initial assessment, Jovana reports experiencing frequent episodes of regurgitation accompanied by stomach discomfort.

How would you go about investigating potential solutions for Jovana?

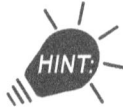

> **HINT:**
>
> Consider investigating the formula's volume and rate of administration, her positioning during and after feeding, and potential gastrointestinal motility issues.

Lina Breik

Commentary

In Jovana's case, managing her nutritional needs while addressing the challenges of spinal muscular atrophy (type 4) requires a thoughtful and individualised approach. Here are some considerations with potential solutions:

1. **Dietary assessment:**
    Begin by conducting a thorough review of Jovana's current nutritional intake, both oral and via the tube. It may be helpful to keep a food-symptoms diary for three days and see if a pattern emerges. Some questions to explore include:

    ▶ How much is she eating orally?

    ▶ Does she need a higher calorie formula to reduce volume administered but maintain the same calorie provision?

    ▶ Does she need a lower calorie formula to avoid overfeeding?

    ▶ Are there specific food items triggering regurgitation or stomach discomfort? It may be the FODMAP content of her food/formula.

2. **Meal timing:**
    Investigate the timing of bolus feeds in relation to her oral intake. Explore whether altering the time of her tube bolus

feeds away from oral mealtimes, or introducing smaller, more frequent bolus feeds, could improve her symptoms.

3. **Bolus administration method:**
   Bolusing 200 ml of a 1.5 kcal/ml formula using a syringe would take around 10–15 minutes. Perhaps that may be too much too fast for Jovanna, especially if she has worsening gastric motility issues. You can explore whether pump feeding a lower calorie formula, such as 1.25 kcal/ml formula at 100 ml/hr for two hours, may be tolerated better.[1]

4. **Tube position check:**
   Ensuring that the PEG tube is properly positioned is another crucial consideration, as misalignment can contribute to her symptoms. This can be checked by liaising with a doctor to order the right type of imaging for her feeding tube.

5. **Gastrointestinal evaluation:**
   Consult with a gastroenterologist to conduct a thorough evaluation of Jovana's gastrointestinal function. This may include procedures like endoscopy, gastric emptying study or other imaging studies to identify any anatomical or functional issues contributing to her symptoms. It may be gastro-oesophageal reflux disease (GORD) or gastroparesis, both of which can be medication managed. It may also be related to faecal impaction where she'll require medication or mechanical support to help her

relieve herself regularly and experience less pressure on her stomach contents.

6. **Speech pathologist consultation:**
Engage a speech pathologist to assess Jovana's swallowing function. The speech pathologist would also evaluate her oral motor skills and explore interventions to improve swallowing coordination, potentially minimising the risk of regurgitation during oral intake. Her feeding position could also be explored and optimised through discussion with the speech pathologist.

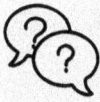

Post-case reflective questions

► How would you approach adjusting Jovana's feeding method to reduce the frequency of regurgitation?

► What non-nutritional factors (e.g. positioning) could help alleviate Jovana's symptoms?

► How would you monitor her progress and assess whether further intervention is needed?

Notes

1. Chen S, Xian W, Cheng S, Zhou C, Zhou H, Feng J, Liu L and Chen L (2015) 'Risk of regurgitation and aspiration in patients infused with different volumes of enteral nutrition'. *Asia Pac Journal of Clinical Nutrition.* 24(2):212-8. doi: 10.6133/apjcn.2015.24.2.12. PMID: 26078237. Available at: https://pubmed.ncbi.nlm.nih.gov/26078237

Case 19

Manuela – Jejunal Feeding

Manuela, a 63-year-old female, underwent a laparoscopic McKeown oesophagectomy for oesophageal cancer. She also had a percutaneous endoscopic jejunostomy (PEJ) inserted in theatre (16 Fr, with a 3 ml water-filled balloon anchoring it in place). Now, she's bravely battling oral chemotherapy to keep the cancer at bay.

Manuela is able to eat a pureed diet through her mouth and is managing three meals daily. Through her feeding tube, she is receiving a 2.0 kcal/ml formula at a rate of 65 ml/hr for 12 hours overnight (2000–0800).

Manuela reports she is experiencing persistent nausea, small vomits overnight and sleep disturbances. A recent endoscopy done by her surgeon revealed no obvious anatomical cause for these symptoms. She is referred to you to determine the next course of action to alleviate her symptoms.

What are some potential considerations and interventions that may alleviate her symptoms?

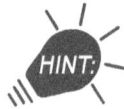

HINT:

Consider investigating the timing and rate of formula administration through the PEJ and potential interactions with oral intake.

Lina Breik

Commentary

Nutrition-related considerations and interventions

1. **Potential overfeeding:**
   Assess if Manuela's oral intake during the day is actually providing adequate nutrition, such that she may not need as much overnight nutrition. Encourage her to titrate up or down her overnight nutrition according to her oral intake to avoid overfeeding. For instance, if Manuela consumes a full dinner plate size of pureed food three times a day, she may not need as much overnight nutrition. Titrating the overnight feeding according to her oral intake may help suppress her symptoms of overnight nausea and vomiting.

2. **Oral meal and pump feed timing:**
   Evaluate the timing of Manuela's overnight feeding in relation to her oral meal schedule. It currently starts at 2000 and stops at 0800, which may be too close to dinner time and breakfast time. Consider adjusting the duration of feeding to better align with her meal times. This may look like increasing the rate of formula per hour so that she would only need 6–8 hours of feeding, rather than 12 hours, thus not cutting into her oral meal times.

3. **Maximum jejunal feeding rate:**

   You may feel uncertain about increasing Manuela's hourly formula volume due to her tube ending in the jejunum. However, evidence supports the titration of jejunal feeds upward without a specified maximum limit.[1,2] There's no substantial clinical evidence supporting the belief that the jejunum can only handle up to 100 ml/hr. In fact, there are documented cases of jejunal boluses being tolerated at rates as high as 300 ml/hr.[1] So, it's essential not to underestimate the jejunum's ability to handle higher volumes in shorter periods of time. Discuss this with Manuela's surgeon to better understand what their understanding is of Manuela's tolerance to a higher pump rate during overnight feeding or larger boluses for daytime feeding.

4. **Daytime bolus feeding:**

   Consider transitioning Manuela to daytime bolus feeding, allowing her to adjust the PEJ bolus based on her oral intake at each meal. This approach could help reduce night-time disturbances. For example, Manuela could be guided to use the PEJ formula as a supplement to her oral intake – if she consumes half of her meal orally, she will then administer half of a PEJ bolus, however, if she manages a full meal, she can skip the PEJ bolus altogether. This flexible feeding strategy would allow her to tailor her nutrition to her needs and comfort, potentially improving her overall well-being.

Other considerations and interventions

1. **Medication side effects:**
    Investigate if Manuela's oral chemotherapy tablets are causing the persistent nausea and vomiting. Consult with her primary doctor to explore alternative medications or adjust the timing of medication administration.

2. **Bowel function optimisation:**
    Ensure Manuela's bowel function is optimised with appropriate aperients and laxatives to alleviate constipation, which may be contributing to her discomfort. Alternatively, you may consult her doctor about the use of a promotility agent to enhance gastric emptying and reduce nausea.

3. **Feeding position:**
    The correct feeding position is for someone to be upright during mealtimes (whether oral or via a tube). However, given her feeds are running overnight, unless medically contraindicated, ensure her bedhead is elevated to at least 30–45 degrees during feeding hours.[3]

4. **PEG-J insertion:**
    As with Sarah's situation in Case 4, a PEG-J tube for Manuela may have the potential to provide some non-invasive decompression therapy to alleviate her symptoms of refractory nausea and vomiting. Close collaboration with

a doctor is needed to determine suitability of this tube for her, if no other intervention works.

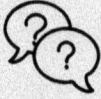

Post-case reflective questions

► What specific considerations are necessary when managing a patient like Manuela on jejunal feeding?

► What signs of intolerance or complications would you monitor closely during her feeding?

Notes

1. Parrish C and Bridges M (2019, April) 'NUTRITION ISSUES IN GASTROENTEROLOGY, SERIES #185. Part III Jejunal Enteral Feeding: The Tail is Wagging the Dog(ma) – Dispelling Myths with Physiology, Evidence, and Clinical Experience'. *Practical Gastroenterology.* [online] Available at: https://med.virginia.edu/ginutrition/wp-content/uploads/sites/199/2019/04/Jejunal-Feeding-Bridges-Parrish-April-2019.pdf

2. Sharma V, Somashekar U, Thakur DS, Kothari R and Sharma D (2022, Jan) 'Prospective randomised trial of bolus vs. continuous regime of jejunostomy feed'. *Tropical Doctor.* 52(1):30-33. doi: 10.1177/00494755211058949. Epub 2021 Nov 20. PMID: 34806486. Available at: https://pubmed.ncbi.nlm.nih.gov/34806486/

3. Serna ED, McCarthy MS. Heads up to prevent aspiration during enteral feeding. Nursing. 2006 Jan;36(1):76-7. doi: 10.1097/00152193-200601000-00058. PMID: 16395034. Available at: https://pubmed.ncbi.nlm.nih.gov/16395034/

Sally – Micronutrients

Meet Sally, a spirited 38-year-old who shares a cosy home with her loving partner. Sally faces the challenge of progressive motor neurone disease, which has led to her reliance on a feeding tube for daily nourishment. This routine has seamlessly woven into her life, providing essential sustenance to support her vibrant spirit.

Sally's feeding regimen consists of 690 ml of a 1.5 kcal/ml commercially made formula per day, administered as three mealtimes: 230 ml at breakfast, 230 ml at lunch and 230 ml at dinner. Between meals, she enjoys pureed snacks orally.

As part of Sally's annual nutritional assessment, her doctor ordered blood tests, which returned with concerning results. Sally's levels of zinc, iron and vitamin C were found to be below optimal ranges – 2.9 umol/L for zinc, 2 umol/L for iron and less than 5 umol/L for vitamin C.

Delving into the composition of Sally's feeding formula, you discover that while the amount she is having (690 ml, 1021 calories) meets 100% of her recommended daily intake (RDI) for zinc and vitamin C, it falls short in providing adequate levels of iron, meeting only 70% of the RDI.

What steps would you take next?

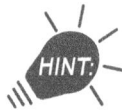

> **HINT:**
>
> Is it a nutrient absorption issue or an intake issue? Consider how you would you go about addressing either of those root causes.

Lina Breik

Commentary

There are two key questions here that can help guide your thinking:

1. Is there a nutrient absorption issue with the zinc and vitamin C given she is meeting 100% of the RDI for both through the formula but her blood test results still appeared deficient?
2. Can the iron deficiency be rectified with added intake or is there an underlying issue contributing to her low iron levels?

Potential next steps

For Zinc and Vitamin C: Sally's doctor could order a stool sample test to check for malabsorption or inflammatory bowel issues which may affect nutrient absorption in the long term.[1] For immediate rectification of the low levels, Sally may benefit from liquid supplementation of each nutrient for a set period of time to address her deficiencies acutely. For example, elemental zinc can be given for 3–4 months to rectify the existing deficiency.[2] It would be necessary to liaise with her doctor before recommending any micronutrient supplementation to ensure it does not interact with any of her existing medications, and to also ensure there is medical oversight for rechecking her nutrient bloods levels after a defined period of supplementation.

For Iron:

1. Incorporate nutrient dense snacks between meals, especially iron rich foods, to complement her feeding tube nutrition.

2. Suggest Sally's doctor consider the following:

   ▶ Administering an intravenous iron infusion or high dose oral supplementation to immediately rectify the deficiency before it worsens.[2]

   ▶ Conducting a menstrual review: Given Sally's low iron levels, it's crucial to assess if menstrual blood loss contributes to her iron deficiency. Sally's doctor can conduct a thorough menstrual review to evaluate the impact on her iron status and discuss potential management strategies.

The key takeaway from Sally's case is that fulfilling 100% of calorie and protein requirements from the tube feeding formula (whether homemade or commercially made) *doesn't guarantee meeting 100% of micronutrient needs.*[3,4]

Advise clients, particularly those at high risk of deficiencies such as the elderly, those receiving nutrition through a jejunal feeding tube, or those post bariatric surgery, to monitor levels annually or more frequently if clinically warranted. [3,4]

Be observant for any clinical signs of micronutrient deficiencies and include them as part of your routine nutritional assessment.[5] Refer to Appendix 2 for a pictorial depiction of the signs to look out for.

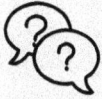

Post-case reflective questions

► How can regular monitoring for micronutrient deficiencies be integrated into care plans for clients who are tube-fed?

► What strategies can help identify and address nutrient malabsorption in clients with deficiencies despite adequate intake?

Notes

1. Azer SA and Sankararaman S (2023, May 16) Steatorrhea. [online] In: StatPearls [Internet]. Treasure Island (FL): StatPearls Publishing. Available at: https://www.ncbi.nlm.nih.gov/books/NBK541055

2. Berger MM, Shenkin A, Dizdar OS, Amrein K, Augsburger M, Biesalski HK, Bischoff SC, Casaer MP, Gundogan K, Lepp H-L, de Man A, Muscogiuri G, Pietka M, Pironi L, Rezzi S, Schweinlin A and Cuerda C (2024) 'ESPEN practical short micronutrient guideline'. *Clinical Nutrition*, 43(3), pp.825–857. doi:https://doi.org/10.1016/j.clnu.2024.01.030. Available at: https://www.clinicalnutritionjournal.com/action/showPdf?pii=S0261-5614%2824%2900041-4

3. Osland EJ, Polichronis K, Madkour R, Watt A and Blake C (2022) 'Micronutrient deficiency risk in long-term enterally fed patients: A systematic review'. *Clinical Nutrition ESPEN*. [online] doi:https://doi.org/10.1016/j.clnesp.2022.09.022. Available at: https://pubmed.ncbi.nlm.nih.gov/36513481/

4. Breik L, Tatucu-Babet OA, Paul E, Duke G, Elliott A, Ridley EJ (2021) 'Micronutrient intake from enteral nutrition in critically ill adult patients: A retrospective observational study'. *Nutrition*. 95:111543. doi: 10.1016/j.nut.2021.111543. Available at: https://www.sciencedirect.com/science/article/abs/pii/S0899900721004056?via%3Dihub

5. Reber E, Gomes F, Vasiloglou MF, Schuetz P and Stanga Z (2019) 'Nutritional Risk Screening and Assessment'. *Journal of Clinical Medicine*, [online] 8(7), p.1065. doi:https://doi.org/10.3390/jcm8071065. Available at: https://www.mdpi.com/2077-0383/8/7/1065

Appendix 1:
Subjective Global Assessment

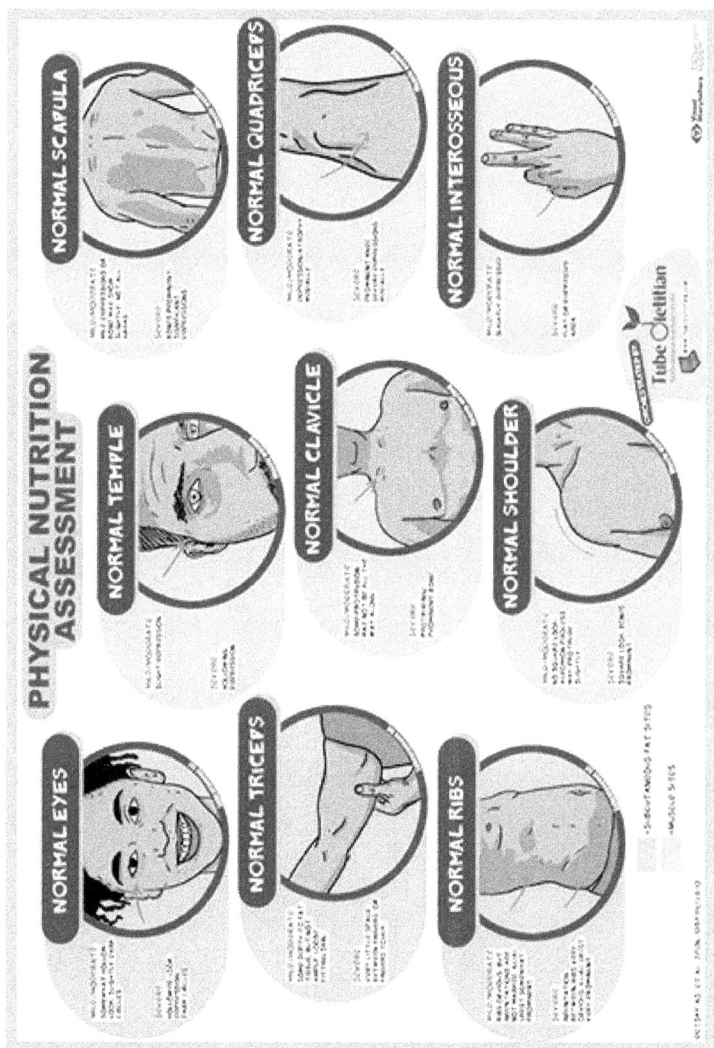

Visit the Tube Dietitian website books page, select the appendix you'd like to download, and enter the code word **TUBE** to access it.

Appendix 2:
Nutrient Deficiency Signs

Visit the Tube Dietitian website books page, select the appendix you'd like to download, and enter the code word **TUBE** to access it.

Acknowledgements

Writing this book has been a rewarding journey, and I am deeply grateful to the individuals and communities who supported me along the way.

To my patients and their families, thank you for sharing your stories, your challenges, and your triumphs with me. Your resilience and strength are the inspiration behind every case in this book. You have taught me that compassionate care goes beyond clinical knowledge and that person-centered care is the true heart of dietetics.

A special thanks to Accredited Practising Dietitian Erin Russell, who took the time to review drafts and provide feedback—your contributions have greatly enhanced the quality of this work.

To my husband, thank you for your unwavering love, patience, and support. You have been my cheerleader through the long nights of writing and editing, and I couldn't have completed this book without your encouragement.

Lastly, thank you to the dietitian community. Your passion for improving the lives of those who rely on feeding tubes is evident in the care you provide each day. I hope this book serves as a resource to further empower you in your important work.

With deep gratitude,

Lina Breik

"So that's what's sad about not eating. The loss of dining, not the loss of food. It may be personal, but for me, unless I'm alone, it doesn't involve dinner if it doesn't involve talking. The food and drink I can do without easily. The jokes, gossip, laughs, arguments and shared memories I miss. Sentences beginning with the words, 'Remember that time?' I ran in crowds where anyone was likely to break out in a poetry recitation at any time. Me too. But not me anymore. So yes, it's sad. Maybe that's why I enjoy this blog. You don't realise it, but we're at dinner right now."

Roger Ebert, Tube-Fed Film Critic (1942–2013)

www.ingramcontent.com/pod-product-compliance
Lightning Source LLC
Chambersburg PA
CBHW040853210326
41597CB00029B/4831